FIFTY SHADES OF
MENOPAUSE

FIFTY SHADES OF MENOPAUSE

Cry, Laugh, Forget...You are not alone!

Mickey Harpaz EdDC

ISBN: 0979334780
ISBN 13: 9780979334788

Disclaimer

This book is intended as a reference volume only, not as a medical manual.

The information given here is designed to help you make informed decisions about your health.

It is not intended as a substitute for any treatment that may have been prescribed by your doctor. If you suspect that you have a medical problem, we urge you to seek competent medical help.

Mention of specific companies, organizations, or authorities in this book does not imply endorsement by the author, nor does mention of specific companies, organizations, or authorities imply that they endorse this book, or its author.

Internet addresses and telephone numbers given in this book were accurate at the time it went to press.

Dedication

*I dedicate the book to the female gender, which has no choice in the matter,
but is brave enough and strong enough to face and confront the challenges
of menopause.
For the women who march toward menopause, parade in it, or walk away from
it...you all deserve more positive insight, patience and compassion.*

Table of Contents

Introduction

Cry, Laugh, Forget...You are not alone!

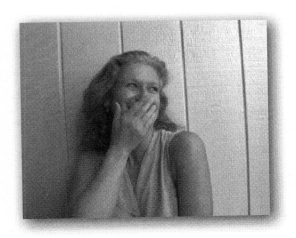

"We are not old. We haven't lost our beauty and we all still hear "Hi There Cutie" and I don't understand why they call it "The Change" everything about me is almost the same."

GWEN A. LEVINE

Almost the same!!!

There are 50 million menopausal women in America and yet, menopause is still considered a taboo topic.

Many women know that it is an inevitable part of life -- a phase that they can't escape, no matter how hard they try -- but they do try to escape it or at best pretend it doesn't exist. After all, no one wants to admit they are getting older; young is in and everyone wants to stay young somehow, but that doesn't stop the clock.

Time marches on. So why not find a way to deal with this elephant in the room? In this age of abundant knowledge at our fingertips and openness about many topics past generations just didn't talk about, we need to start talking about menopause.

However, understanding...**you are not alone**...the journey maybe shorter, or maybe longer! The symptoms may vary! The frequency and severity may be a piece of a cake...or may come as tornado forces...just one thought to follow...you are **not alone!** And guess what? **You are not crazy either...It is Menopause.**

"I was going to be outside mowing the grass, and since my husband calls me during the day, I wanted to leave a message on our answering machine letting him know what I was doing. My cell phone was in my car in the garage. I went to my car, leaving the back door of the house open, and dialed my home phone number. Suddenly I heard the phone ringing inside the house. I jumped out of the car, ran inside and answered the phone!! I even got angry because SOMEONE hung up after only one ring. I then went BACK out to my car to call me again! When I began dialing my number, I realized what I had done. I just sat in my car in the garage and laughed and laughed." P. M.

"One day I was scrambling in my purse looking for my cell phone - while I was talking on my cell phone! I frantically pulled out my wadded ball of Kleenex, an old lipstick, my wallet, my sunglasses case and my glasses case before I said to the other person: Hold on, I can't find my cell phone." D. R.

"There was the time I went to the store for Bleach, Apples and Gas. Memory abbreviation= BAG. Guess what? I came home with a new pocketbook..." D. L.

"After reporting to police that my car had been stolen, I had gone to Rent-a-Car, so I could drive to work that coming Monday morning. On my way back from the place...what did I spot, but my forlorn little car, sitting in front of the beauty parlor, where I had left it (and walked home from instead of driving it home.... duh). Just imagine my horror at what I had done. I'm still shocked that I did it. The worst part, was calling the police back again, and having to tell them, what I had done...Not to mention...the insurance company...God help me" S.G.

"I was changing clothes in front of my 3 year old granddaughter, trying to be as discrete about it as possible, especially since her new interest is in the human body. Well she was pointing to my breast and asked, "What's that?" I replied, "Honey, that's my breasts." "Well" she said, "They sure are long." M.A.

You probably noticed or previously heard that Menstruation, Menopause and Mental breakdowns are all women's problems begin with MEN. So, ladies time to take care of that.

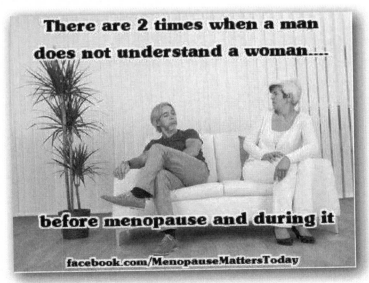

"11 Things My Husband Needs To Know About Menopausal Me" by Michelle Combs, couldn't address this matter in a better way:

"A menopausal GPS for his upcoming trip.
Keep your stupid menopause jokes to yourself…
Tropical moments don't mean we're on vacation…
No, I don't hate you, but my hormones really dislike you…
Don't take it personally, ___hole…
Understanding goes a long way…
Don't expect logic, Mr. Spock…
Stop humping my leg…
Boobs are now a grope-free zone…
Why yes, I'm developing the "old lady odor"…
Turn up the fan high and pray for a polar vortex…
There's a storm a comin'…"

The History of Menopause

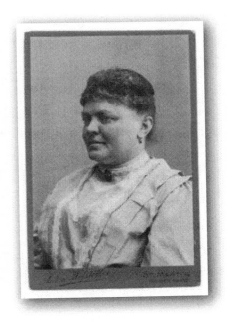

Menopause had been viewed as a disease in the last 100 years. Women have been experiencing menopause for eons for as long as there have been women on planet earth.

A review of the history of menopause may put your own trials and tribulations with menopause into a perspective that may be helpful to you.

Earliest known references to what we now call menopause, occurred during the ancient Greek civilization....approximately 2,500 years ago.

Mickey Harpaz EdDC

Aristotle wrote of menopause, without calling it that. He noted that women stop giving birth after the age of 40. The word menopause itself comes from the Greek, 'men' for month, and 'pausis' for pause. (260)

The next significant reference to what we now call menopause, occurred in the 13th century.

Trotula of Salerno, who may have been a female physician, wrote a book called The Diseases of Women. (261) Here is a translation of a reference to menopause:

"Since in women not so much heat abounds that is suffices to use up the moistures which daily collect in them, their weakness cannot endure so much exertion as to be able to put forth that moisture to the outside air as in the case of men.

Nature herself, on account of this deficiency, has assigned for them a special purgation namely the menses, commonly called flowers. Now a purgation of this sort usually befalls women about the 13th or 14th year or a little later according to whether heat or cold abounds in them more.

It lasts up to about the 50th year if she is lean; sometimes up to the 60th or 65th year if she is moist; in the moderately fat up to about the 45th."

Until the 18th century, menopause was usually perceived as a natural phenomenon. The prevailing mindset about women's physical conditions was that they had to do with body fluids. This changed in the 19th century.

Dr. Charles Négrier is credited with being the first person to use the term menopause in 1821. Instead of pointing to bodily fluids to explain women's physical conditions, the new trend was to attribute them to body organs. (262)

Because women were complaining of depression, hot flashes, and irregular periods, doctors were quick to diagnoses these women with "hysteria", a term that literally referred to the uterus in Latin.

The Greek word 'hysterus' means womb, thus, the uterus literally caused 'hysteria'. The uterus was thought to be the organ responsible for physical problems that led to **neuroses.**

In the 1850's, Edward Tilt, MD determined that "the keystone of mental pathology" was the uterus. By 1870, the surgical procedure of hysterectomy was perfected as a quick method to deal with menopausal complaints.

In 1902, English physiologists Ernest Starling and William Bayliss discovered the first-ever hormone. (264)

It was called secretin and it helped maintain water homeostasis throughout the body. This discovery was a significant milestone in gaining a better understanding of menopause as a whole.

Then in 1925, modern scientists unveiled human hormonal make-up and were able to differentiate between estrogen and progesterone. In the 1930s people started describing menopause as a deficiency disease.

Over the next few decades there would be increased discoveries of how to use estrogen to help deal with a variety of physical and emotional symptoms associated with menopause. These findings have led to the "medicalization" of menopause.

THE MEDICALIZATION OF MENOPAUSE

If menopause is not a disease, why do doctors treat it with drugs?

Is menopause a disease or a natural condition?

If it is a disease, it seems natural that doctors would treat it with drugs to try to cure it. If it is a natural condition, it raises a question about whether doctors should be using drugs for it at all.

In March 2005, the National Institutes of Health (NIH) issued a statement saying that menopause is (264) but rather a natural part of life, just like puberty. It called for the de-medicalization of menopause. (265)

Definition: *"Medicalization is a social process through which a human experience or condition is culturally defined as pathological and treatable as a medical condition."* (266)

Yet today, the medical profession is not regarding menopause as it regards puberty, or even menstruation.

The favored solution offered by mainstream medicine, for complaints about menopause symptoms, is hormone therapy … a drug solution.

How did menopause become medicalized?

- The medicalization of menopause began with the discovery of estrogen in 1923, by Dr Edgar Allen, and the discovery of progesterone in 1933.

Estrogen was first approved by the FDA as a treatment for menopause in 1942, despite the fact that, Dr Edgar Allen published a paper in the journal Cancer Research saying that his most recent research showed estrogen to be a carcinogen. (267)

- Estrogen therapy (HRT) really began to take off in the 1960s. In 1966, Robert Wilson, MD, published a book entitled "Feminine Forever".

Dr Wilson called menopause a "living decay" during which women descended into a "vapid cow-like" state.

By giving estrogen, Dr. Wilson claimed, he could magically transform a "dull cow" into a supple, younger-looking wife.

It became a best seller. Women were going to doctors and demanding "the pills that will keep me from growing old". (268)

- In 1970 the Senate conducted an investigation into birth control pill side effects. At one of the hearings an expert said "Estrogen is to cancer what fertilizer is to wheat".

Despite this, the hormone's chief manufacturer, Wyeth Pharmaceuticals, next launched an aggressive marketing campaign. A 1975 ad read, "Almost any tranquilizer might calm her down… but at her age, estrogen may be what she really needs"

- Over the next two decades, drug companies changed their advertisements to scientific-sounding arguments for the virtues of hormone replacement.

There are a growing number of people who think that pharmaceutical companies invent diseases to enable them to sell cures in their never ending pursuit of profits. (269)

Doctors used these arguments to convince their menopausal patients that taking estrogen, and later estrogen together with progestin, would not only decrease their hot flashes but also reduce their risk of heart disease and cancer.

Millions of American women believed them!

- As doctors are not trained in menopause, they were taught about the virtues of estrogen therapy by pharmaceutical companies. (203)

  Pharmaceutical companies promote and run medical conventions and conferences to promote their products. They offer doctors attractive gifts and these are normally the products doctors have information about and are educated in, making them the ones they prescribe to their patients. (225,226)
- Dr Kent Holtorf, MD, has suggested that societies such as The Endocrine Society, The North American Menopause Society and The American College of Obstetricians and Gynecologists have allowed themselves to be influenced by significant relationships with the pharmaceutical companies. (270)
- One gynecologist has stated "As a board certified, OB/GYN trained at Emory University, I am embarrassed by what I learned in residency concerning hormone physiology.

  It is a crime that this information is not taught in residencies. Instead we are bombarded by propaganda and misinformation by the so-called leaders in our field"
- Dr Susan Love, MD, a noted cancer researcher, said in a New York Times editorial that there was a lot of scientific theorizing about the benefits of HRT, but very little scientific research. (271)

  "What happened is that medical practice, as it so often does, got ahead of medical science. We made observations and developed hypotheses — and then forgot to prove them."

This is how menopause became medicalized, and **still is medicalized today**; despite the 2005 statement by the NIH that menopause should be de-medicalized.

Menopause: What May Lie Ahead For You

Some women describe menopause as a roller coaster ride. They experience mental, emotional and physical ups and downs over a period of years. For other women, menopause is a downhill ride into the bowels of hell.

Most women would love to know when menopause will end ... or at least have a way to predict the progression of symptoms. The former is not known. The latter is known.

Although much is still not known about menopause, the cause of the symptoms you are experiencing is known for certain. Your symptoms are caused by a change in the relative levels of the hormones in your body, from their levels prior to perimenopause.

This change is started by changes in the levels of estrogen and progesterone at the onset of perimenopause. Changes in the levels of estrogen and progesterone, triggers changes in the levels of other hormones in your body.

The levels of your hormones are changing on an ongoing basis for years, as you progress through the different stages of menopause.

It is not as if they change from one level to another and remain at the new level. The levels keep changing as you go from one menopause stage to the next.

STAGES OF MENOPAUSE

There is a road map that identifies the different stages of menopause, which is called, Stages of Reproductive Aging Workshop (STRAW).

It can help you to identify the stage you are in now and it can help you to predict what comes next in your progression through menopause.

Reproductive aging in women is a natural progression through 3 stages: reproduction, the menopausal transition (perimenopause), and post menopause.

The reproductive stage has three sub-stages, early, middle and late. Menopause transition has two sub-stages, early and late. Post menopause has two sub-stages, early and late.

The reproductive stage begins when a women starts to menstruate.....this is at 12 years old on average. It ends with the onset of perimenopause....for most women this is in their forties. While hormone levels oscillate during these years ... during the menstrual cycle and during pregnancy ... they stay in the same general levels relative to one another.

For most of the time during the perimenopause stages, estrogen levels are high and fluctuating while progesterone levels are falling. The ratios between them and other hormones are changing from what they were in the reproductive stages. (7)

In post menopause stages, estrogen and progesterone settle at low levels and remain there. Other hormone levels tend to normalize.

Two sub-stages of perimenopause:

1. Early perimenopause is marked by increased variability in menstrual cycle length. Your cycles may shorten to 24 to 27 days instead of 28 to 31, and your periods might be heavier or lighter than they used to be. (272)

While estrogen levels will fluctuate, in general they will be approximately 30% higher than they were during reproductive stages. Progesterone levels will be falling from the levels they were at during reproductive stages.

You will experience menopause symptoms increasingly. Breast tenderness, mood swings, fluid retention, weight gain, migraine headaches, disturbed sleep and premenstrual symptoms are common. Hot flashes occur increasingly.

2. Late perimenopause is marked by hit or miss ovulation. This stage is characterized by two or more skipped menstrual cycles. Just when you think you will never have a period again, your period may come back. (273)

Your estrogen levels will continue to fluctuate and remain high during the first part of this stage.

As you progress through this stage toward post menopause, estrogen will fall to very low levels. Progesterone will fall to even lower levels than in the early perimenopause stage.

You may experience any of the full range of menopause symptoms. Hot flashes and night sweats will occur more frequently and will be more intense as you approach post menopause. (274)

POST MENOPAUSE STAGES:
Early post menopause is characterized by the following changes:

- No more periods.
- Hot flashes and night sweats will be more frequent and more intense than during any other stage of menopause.
- Vaginal dryness and discomfort is common during this stage.
- Many women experience a decrease in the symptoms they had been experiencing in perimenopause.
- Estrogen and progesterone levels will be low and remain low.
- Other hormone levels will begin to normalize.

Late post menopause is characterized by fewer and less intense hot flashes and night sweats. They will disappear, or reduce to insignificance, for most women.

Most other symptoms will disappear as well. Vaginal dryness and discomfort will remain. This symptom only improves with treatment.

Unfortunately it is not possible to say how long each of the stages of menopause will last.

Just as every woman experiences menopause differently, the amount of time in each stage varies from woman to woman. Some women pass through all stages in 1-2 years. For others, it can take 20 years or longer.

Increased knowledge of the stages of menopause should enable you to better predict what lies ahead and to manage it better.

How to effectively manage your progression through the stages of menopause?

1. Eliminate all processed and junk foods from your diet. These foods exacerbate your symptoms. Adopt a diet that is based on eating fresh foods when possible. i.e. – unprocessed meat, fish, milk, eggs, legumes, fruits, grains and vegetables.
2. Engage in at least 30 minutes of aerobic activity/exercise every day.
3. Manage your level of stress during menopause by doing a technique that reduces stress. Stress exacerbates symptoms during every stage of menopause.
4. Re-balance your hormones. The most effective way to do this is to get the levels of your hormones tested and then re-balanced. However this is a costly option and may be beyond the financial means of many women. There will be lab fees (hundreds of dollars) to test your hormone levels and physician fees to help you re-balance them. Often, this is not covered by health insurance policies.

A safe, effective and inexpensive way to relieve your perimenopause symptoms is to use a self-administered natural progesterone cream. Natural progesterone cream will increase your progesterone level and reduce your estrogen levels. (Will be discussed later in the book)

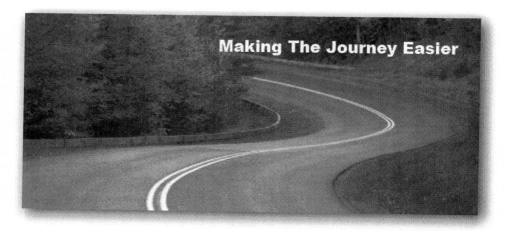

If you search the internet for advice about how to make your menopause journey easier, you will find an abundance of advice about changing/improving your lifestyle....including:

- Healthy eating – this means basing your diet around foods rich in natural vitamins and minerals. It also means eliminating/reducing junk foods from your diet.
- Eliminating/reducing your intake of caffeine.
- Eliminating/reducing your intake of alcohol.
- Daily exercise.
- Regular use of a stress reduction technique to reduce your stress.

There is no doubt that if you do all of these things, your menopause journey will be easier than if you don't do them. Collectively they help to reduce the severity and frequency of menopause symptoms.

Chances are that you already know this. Many menopausal women are doing these things, yet are still experiencing debilitating menopause symptoms.

For these women, what is missing from the advice above?

Three things are missing from the advice above, which will help you to have an easier menopause journey:

1. Understanding the cause of menopause symptoms.
2. Finding a treatment/remedy that relieves menopause symptoms.
3. Managing expectations about menopause symptoms and the duration of menopause.

If you have adopted the lifestyle changes recommended above, your next step in making your menopause journey easier is to understand the cause of menopause symptoms.

UNDERSTANDING THE CAUSE OF MENOPAUSE SYMPTOMS

The hormone levels in your body change radically with the onset of perimenopause, from their levels prior to it. This is the cause of all of your menopause symptoms.

Prior to perimenopause, all of the hormones in your body work in harmony by co-existing with one another in a certain ratio. Your hormones are said to be balanced. During perimenopause, not only do the levels of your hormones change, but the ratios between them change as well. Your hormones are said to be un-balanced.

All of the hormonal changes in your body during menopause are triggered by changes in the levels of estrogen and progesterone.

While estrogen levels are generally falling during perimenopause, they are fluctuating. This means that their levels go up and down. They surge and fall cyclically. Progesterone levels are consistently falling throughout perimenopause.

This means that the ratio between estrogen and progesterone changes from what it was prior to perimenopause. There is more estrogen in your body, relative to progesterone. Or, in other words, there is **insufficient progesterone** in your body. (1)

During post menopause your body makes a very small amount of estrogen. It makes zero progesterone.

TREATMENTS/REMEDIES THAT RELIEVE MENOPAUSE SYMPTOMS

There are 3 categories of treatments/remedies that have helped women to relieve their symptoms:

1. Natural treatments and remedies – these include natural herbs, vitamin and mineral supplements, and treatments such as acupuncture, hypnosis, and Chinese Medicine etc. (237)

These treatments have provided relief to some women but not all women, and for some symptoms, but not all symptoms.

These treatments/remedies do not address the imbalance between estrogen and progesterone that triggers the changes in the levels and ratios of all of the hormones in your body.

These treatments/remedies appeal to women who are averse to taking synthetic drugs to relieve their symptoms.

2. Conventional HRT – This is the treatment recommended by most physicians. (275)

It consists of taking synthetic estrogen or estrogen + progestin (a synthetic chemical that resembles progesterone, but is not progesterone, and it does not do what progesterone does in your body).

Conventional HRT increases the level of estrogen in your body. It does not increase the level of progesterone.

Synthetic estrogen and progestin is not identical to the estrogen and progesterone made by your body. Therefor your body responds differently to them than it does to the hormones made by your body.

Conventional HRT provides effective relief from hot flashes, night sweats and vaginal atrophy/dryness. It does not provide relief from mental and emotional menopause symptoms.

Medical studies have found that conventional HRT increases the risk of breast cancer and stroke. Because of this, doctors recommend that it be taken for under 5 years. (Will be discussed later)

Studies have found that many women experience hot flashes for approximately 10 years. If a woman stops taking conventional HRT after 5 years, she is likely to re-experience the symptoms she had prior to taking it. (Will be discussed later)

Conventional HRT does not address the imbalance between estrogen and progesterone that triggers the changes in the levels and ratios of all of the hormones in your body, and therefore, it does not address the cause of menopause symptoms.

3. Bioidentical hormone replacement – these are natural hormones that are identical to the hormones made by your body. Your body responds to them in the same way it does to the hormones that are made by your body. (196)

Taking bioidentical hormones replacement, effectively relieves mental and emotional symptoms, as well hot flashes, night sweats and vaginal atrophy.

It addresses the imbalance between estrogen and progesterone and the other hormones in your body. It is the only treatment that addresses the imbalances in these hormones.

There is no known health risks associated with taking bioidentical hormones. Therefore, unlike conventional HRT, you can take bioidentical hormones for as long as you are experiencing symptoms.

Focus On Making Your Menopause Journey Better ... Not On When It Will End

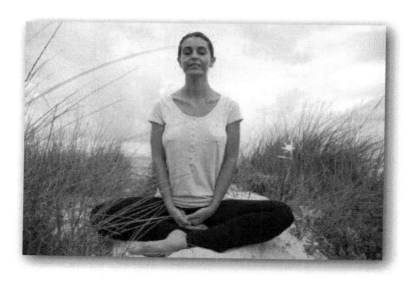

"It is good to have an end to journey toward; but it is the journey that matters, in the end"

ERNEST HEMINGWAY

When will it end?
I wish I had a dollar for each time I have been asked this question. I would be wealthy today.

There is no way of knowing when your journey will end. Just as every person is absolutely unique, so is every journey through menopause absolutely unique.

I want to share with you some thoughts of Roseanne Barr about the menopause journey. She is on the other side now:

"You can bet that a realist like moi isn't here to take up your time pretending that menopause is a walk in the park.

I've heard that close to a third of women find menopause to be, at worst, a temporary and fairly inconsequential passage. To those women, I'd like to say: congratulations, and I hate you!

My experience was a raw and often torturous ordeal."

When you're going through menopause it can seem like a never ending battle. You may be experiencing a frustrating pattern, where just when you think you're over the worst of it, the symptoms come back stronger and knock you back down again.

It can be demoralizing and it's common to wonder whether the battle will ever be over.

While it may sometimes feel like a "forever" experience, for 99.5% of women it will not be a forever experience. Their menopause journey will end.

However approximately 5 women out of every 1,000 women may experience some symptoms for the rest of their lives...but their symptoms later in life will be milder than previously.

THE SPECTRUM OF MENOPAUSE JOURNEYS
Just as some women experience mild menopause symptoms throughout their journey, while others experience moderate or severe symptoms, the length of the journey for each woman varies.

Some women complete their journey in:

1. 1-2 years
2. 6-10 years
3. 11-20 years
4. More than 20 years

Some women experience a short perimenopause and a long post menopause. Other women experience a long perimenopause and a short post menopause.

Some women experience a short menopause journey, but have severe symptoms throughout it. Other women may experience a longer menopause journey, but with mild to moderate symptoms.

Some women may experience mild to moderate perimenopause symptoms, but more severe symptoms during post menopause. Other women may experience severe symptoms during perimenopause, but mild to moderate symptoms in post menopause.

Every woman is different. Every menopause journey is different. Some of the factors that influence the timing and experience of menopause are

- Genetics
- Lifestyle
- Diet
- Stress
- General health
- Cultural perspective

The advice I give to my menopausal women patients:

1. Educate yourself about the stages of menopause and the phases of perimenopause.

This will give you some idea about where you are in the menopause journey and what may lie ahead.

2. Become more physically active.
3. Eat properly, on time, and fresh non-process foods.
4. Adopt a stress reduction technique and do it regularly.

Some examples are meditation, yoga, and relaxation therapy. For others it can be walks in a peaceful setting. Still others may find that listening to calming music reduces their stress.

5. Educate yourself about the all of the various treatments/remedies that can relieve menopause symptoms.

Adopt one of the treatments/remedies that make the most sense to you. If it relieves your symptoms, stick with it.

If that treatment/remedy is not working for you, adopt another treatment/remedy that makes sense to you.

Persist and you will find a treatment/remedy that will make your journey through menopause easier.

6. Stay focused on 1-5 above. Do not allow you attention to become riveted on when your menopause journey will end.

What to Expect After Menopause?

Much has been written about perimenopause and menopause (that point in time when a woman has had 12 consecutive months without a period).

If you are in perimenopause, or approaching it, and you have questions about what to expect as you progress through perimenopause to menopause, the STRAW system may answer many of your questions.

Too little has been written about post menopause (the period of time after menopause) and today, most women spend at least one-third of their lives after menopause (276). Many women are wondering about what to expect after menopause.

If you are expecting your symptoms to vanish when you reach menopause, you may be disappointed. In most cases, women gradually stop feeling symptoms. Unfortunately, that is not always the case.

During post menopause, hormone levels may continue to fluctuate, bringing with them symptoms you are already familiar with and new symptoms that you may not have experienced during perimenopause. Also, some of the symptoms you experienced during perimenopause may intensify.

Some of the more common post menopause symptoms are hot flashes, vaginal atrophy, loss of libido, insomnia, weight gain, and joint aches and pains.

Before providing some detail about these symptoms, it may be helpful to first discuss what happens to your sex hormones during post menopause.

Your sex hormones are responsible for post menopause symptoms, just as they are responsible for premenopausal symptoms.

WHAT HAPPENS TO YOUR HORMONES DURING POST MENOPAUSE?

- Estrogen – perimenopause is characterized by fluctuating estrogen levels. In post menopause, estrogen levels bottom out and stay low. About 6 months before menopause, estrogen levels drop significantly. (276)
- Estrogen levels continue to fall during post menopause, but not to zero. While your ovaries no longer produce estrogen, your body makes estrogen in other ways.
- Progesterone – progesterone levels fall more than estrogen levels. While your ovaries no longer produce progesterone, your adrenal glands produce a very small amount of progesterone
- Testosterone – in postmenopausal women, testosterone production falls, but does not decrease as much as estrogen and progesterone.

This can cause testosterone levels to be higher relative to the other female sex hormones, sometimes leading postmenopausal women to have deeper voices or more noticeable facial hair.

The 6 most common post menopause symptoms:

1. Hot flashes tend to be more intensive for the first 2 years after menopause, than they are during perimenopause.

   Experts don't know exactly why this happens, but it's believed to be related to the hypothalamus, the portion of the brain that regulates temperature. The hypothalamus is acutely sensitive to estrogen levels.

2. Vaginal atrophy is a treatable chronic condition that affects the vagina and the surrounding tissues during and after menopause, due to declining levels of estrogen. (86)

Symptoms include vaginal dryness, pain and bleeding during intercourse, itching in and around the vagina, vaginal soreness, urinary tract infections and painful urination.

It affects over 50% of postmenopausal women, but few talk about it. It does not improve by itself and it gets worse over time, if it is not treated.

3. Many women experience a decrease in libido during perimenopause. That decrease intensifies after menopause.

One survey of 580 postmenopausal women, conducted by Siecus – the Sexuality Information and Education Council of the United States, found that 45 percent of the women reported a decrease in sexual desire after menopause, 37 percent reported no change and 10 percent reported an increase. (95)

It is caused by a fall in estrogen levels and testosterone during post menopause. Falling estrogen levels brings on vaginal atrophy, which affects libido. Decreased testosterone directly reduces libido.

4. The Sleep Foundation reports that 61% of postmenopausal women experience insomnia. (10) Insomnia in postmenopausal women is caused by decreasing hormone levels and aging.

Decreasing levels of estrogen causes a decrease in the hormone serotonin, which is used to create melatonin – a sleep hormone. Progesterone works to induce sleep, but it is decreasing during post menopause.

Another Sleep Foundation study has found that the postmenopausal age group is more prone to insomnia than all younger female age groups. (15)

5. Postmenopausal women are prone to weight gain and storing fat around the stomach.

Many studies have found that the loss of estrogen leads to insulin resistance, which results in increased fat storage and difficulty losing weight. Also, the metabolism slows down with aging. If you do not alter your diet and exercise more, you are prone to weight gain. (Will be discussed later)

6. 57% of postmenopausal women, who were two years beyond menopause, said that they experience significant joint pain. (140)

This is not surprising, because joint pain is associated with inflammation. Estrogen acts as an anti-inflammatory and estrogen levels are low during post menopause.

I will go into much more detail about each of the above post menopause symptoms in future posts and I will discuss what you can do to relieve each of them.

Many women have said that, after post menopause symptoms abate, post menopause is one of the best periods of their lives. You can look forward to this.

Finally, I would be remiss if I didn't mention that postmenopausal women are at increased risk of osteoporosis and cardiovascular disease.

Low levels of estrogen weaken bones. The National Institute of Aging says that half of American women over the age of 50 will probably have a bone break or fracture later in life because of osteoporosis. (227)

An overall increase in cardiovascular disease among women is seen about 10 years after menopause.

It is believed that low levels of estrogen contribute to this. Estrogen is believed to have a positive effect on the inner layer of artery wall, helping to keep blood vessels flexible. That means they can relax and expand to accommodate blood flow. (278)

Neither osteoporosis nor cardiovascular disease is inevitable. There are steps you can take to reduce your risk of these diseases.

Is Society At Large Becoming More Aware About Menopause?

Summer may be coming to a close, but for women dealing with hot flashes, night sweats, and the other entire menopause symptoms, things aren't cooling down just yet.

But it does bring us to the month of September, the month that Congress declared to be national menopause awareness month.

The intention of having a national menopause awareness month is to draw the attention of the public at large to the challenges faced by menopausal women.

It is also to reinforce that women and their health care providers must have accurate, unbiased menopause-related information to make informed decisions that will lead to improved health and quality of life both around menopause and beyond.

While progress has been made in making menopause less of a taboo subject than it has been, many women still feel uncomfortable talking openly about menopause and its symptoms.

I know this because I receive frequent requests from women asking me to turn my Facebook page, which is a public page, into a private page.

They say that they do not want their friends to know about their menopause and the symptoms that they are experiencing.

MENOPAUSE AWARENESS IN DOCTORS

Menopause is still not understood by most doctors. It was just 2 years ago that Johns Hopkins Medical School conducted a study of more than 500 ob-gyn resident doctors, across America, to determine the training ob-gyns receive in menopause matters. (203)

They found that:

- Only 20% of the ob-gyn residents had received formal training in their ob-gyn curriculum in regard to menopause matters.
- Just 15% of the ob-gyn residents had received practical training to help you with issues that you are facing during menopause.

The lead author of the study, Mindy S. Christianson, a clinical fellow in the Division of Reproductive Endocrinology and Infertility in the Department of Gynecology and Obstetrics at the Johns Hopkins University School of Medicine said:

"It's clear from the results that the residents who responded admit that their knowledge and clinical management skills of menopause medicine are inadequate."

If just 15% of ob-gyn residents have received practical training in menopause, what do you think is the likelihood that your GP has received any training at all in menopause?

What is the likelihood that he/she will be able to provide you with menopause help?

An earlier study of ob-gyn residents found that most residents did not feel comfortable managing menopause patients with 75.8% reporting feeling "barely comfortable" and 8.4% feeling "not at all comfortable." (279)

Given the findings of these studies, it is not surprising that a majority of menopausal women do not feel that their doctors are helping them to overcome their menopause issues.

I constantly hear the following types of complaints from women about what their doctor has said when they talk to their doctors about their symptoms:

- Your blood work is normal....it can't be menopause.
- You are too young.
- You're depressed....just take these antidepressants.
- It's all in your head.
- Every woman goes through menopause. Millions of women before you have survived it. You too will survive it.
- Menopause is not life threatening. Get a grip!

HOWEVER, SOME PROGRESS HAS BEEN MADE TO HELP DOCTORS HELP YOU:

While it is too soon to expect the medical establishment to have corrected the education it provides to doctors about menopause, such that it translates into real help being provided to menopausal women, some progress is being made to provide doctors with more information about menopause.

- The North American Menopause Society (NAMS) has recognized this gap in the training of doctors. It has developed a menopause competency examination. (280)

    All licensed healthcare providers (including doctors, nurses, and physician assistants) are eligible to sit for this examination. Those who pass this rigorous competency examination have demonstrated their expertise in the field and are awarded the credential of NCMP, which stands for NAMS Certified Menopause Practitioner.
- There is a directory of menopause healthcare providers, on the NAMS site, that will help you find doctors who understand menopause. Just enter your zip code and the search results will reveal doctors in your vicinity. (281)

It is advisable to tick the box that limits the search results to NCMP practitioners, because the NAMS directory also contains details of doctors who do not have the NCMP credential.

- A new tool has just been developed to equip doctors with fundamental information about menopause that will help them to diagnose and manage your symptoms.

The tool is called The Practitioner Toolkit for Managing the Menopause. (282) It includes a diagnostic tool, as well as a compendium of approved hormone and non-hormonal therapies.

The tool is provided free of charge for doctors…. anywhere in the world. It includes a flow chart of standardized questions for doctors to ask, and assess women who are potentially experiencing menopause.

It also flags safety concerns and provides a list of all hormone therapies approved by regulators in different countries and lists non-hormonal therapies that have evidence to support their use.

MENOPAUSE AWARENESS IN SOCIETY AT LARGE

There is still much to do to increase menopause awareness in society at large. Many women still talk about intolerance:

1. From their husbands and partners concerning menopause matters.
2. In the workplace to their menopause issues.
3. From friends who experience no or mild symptoms.

To achieve a noticeable increase in menopause awareness in society at large is going to take time. After all, women have been experiencing menopause since the beginning of human life on earth.

Let's use menopause awareness month – this year and in subsequent years – to try to achieve a noticeable increase in awareness about menopause in our lifetime. If we do not achieve it in our lifetime, we can at least make it better for our daughters!

How to Get More Help from Your Doctor

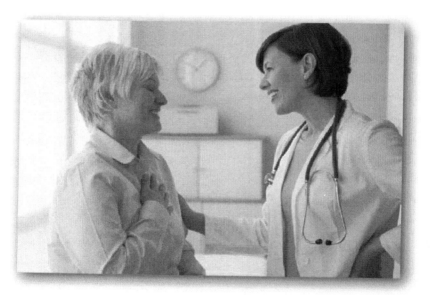

Bad experiences with doctors abound from menopausal women. Some common complaints from menopausal women are:

- My doctor doesn't understand menopause.
- My doctor doesn't listen to me.
- My doctor just shoves me off.
- My doctor is just a pill pusher.
- My doctor doesn't care.

Almost all such complaints are due to two main factors:

- Most doctors do not understand menopause.
- Doctors spend too little time with a patient during a patient's visit.

As discussed in the previous chapter, and in summary, a Johns Hopkins Medical School study found that more than 80% of gynecologists have received no formal training in menopause. 85% of them feel uncomfortable dealing with menopausal patients.

If gynecologists have not been trained in menopause, what is the likelihood that your primary care physician has been trained in menopause?!

WHY THE AMOUNT OF TIME YOU GET WITH YOUR DOCTOR IS SO SHORT?

Some researchers have found that patients have an average of only 8-10 minutes per appointment with their doctors.

However, a survey of more than 15,000 physicians in the United States found that, on average, a physician sees each patient for 13 to 16 minutes.

Whether the correct figure is 8-10 minutes or 13-16 minutes per patient visit, the amount of time a doctor spends with a patient is too little.

In the United States, doctors are not paid according to the amount of time they spend with the patient. They are incentivized to see as many patients as possible and to do as many procedures as possible. This means spending as little time as possible with each patient.

Doctors are paid by insurance companies and Medicare according to the number of patients they see and the number of procedures they perform for patients. Their pay is fixed per procedure. If they spend a long time with a patient doing a particular procedure, or a short time, their pay is the same. (283)

If a doctor takes too long doing a particular procedure, it costs him/her money. If they take less than the prescribed time to do the procedure, they will have extra time to do something else that can make them more money.

If you ever feel as if your doctor is in a hurry to end your visit, this is the reason.

HOW THE SYSTEM OF RECOMPENSE FOR DOCTORS AFFECTS DOCTORS AND YOU?

Most people who want to become a doctor have an altruistic motive. They want to help people. They are empathetic, which is a key quality to have if you want to help people.

Studies have shown that their empathy wanes often before they complete their training. (284) Young doctors often work 80 hours a week.

They are given targets for the number of patients they must see in a day, by profit minded medical organizations. One study revealed that interns spend on average of just 8 minutes with a patient.

By the time they complete their training and enter into medical practice, many have lost their positive outlook on the practice of medicine. Not long after entering into practice, they may feel the stress associated with the system that requires them to curtail time spent with patients in order to realize income needs.

They may become impatient, occasionally indifferent, at times dismissive or paternalistic to patients. They may interrupt patients when they are talking to save time and bring the patients visit to an earlier conclusion.

This has led to an increasing number of doctors who talk about "burnout" as a result of practicing medicine, (285) unhappy doctors and obviously unhappy and discontent patients.

WHAT TO DO TO IMPROVE THE CARE YOU GET FROM YOUR DOCTOR?

Dr. Leana Wen, MD and author of the book *"When Doctors Don't Listen"*, has some tips that will help you to manage your meetings with your doctor and get answers to the questions you have (286):

1. Open with "I need a partnership…" or "Let's work together to figure out the best journey for me."
2. Talk more about your STORY (and less about your SYMPTOMS). You might have 20 symptoms that can send your doctor's head spinning. Use the narrative to tell your story – what is your everyday experience and how/why it is affecting you.
3. Ask about your diagnosis. Be prepared to question, clarify and paraphrase. "What are you recommending?" "Why is this best route for me?" "Who will be calling me back?" "What do you hope the tests will show us?" "What are our next steps?"

ALSO, THE FOLLOWING CAN BE DONE:

- Be mindful of your doctor's limited time.
- Prepare for your appointment. Be concise about your symptoms and stick to facts. You want your doctor to receive all the important information about your symptoms. Carefully prepare any questions you would like answered.

An organized approach can allow your doctor more time to answer all your questions.

- If your doctor interrupts you when you are describing your symptoms or asking a question, interrupt your doctor!

Doctors have learned to interrupt patients when they are talking, to reduce the time of the visit. Studies have shown that it takes only 23 seconds before a doctor interrupts the patient. (284, 285)

If your doctor interrupts you, you can hold up your hand in a way that tells your doctor to stop and to listen to you. Politely ask your doctor to listen to all of your symptoms, or to let you ask your entire question.

- If your doctor uses words or concepts you do not understand, interrupt him/her. Ask your doctor to explain it in lay terms. This will help you to come away from your visit having learned what you need to know.

And, now I believe you are ready for the Fifty Shades of Menopause.

The Fifty Shades of Menopause

"Above all, be the heroine of your life, not the victim."

NORA EPHRON

Fatigue Is So Bad ... Some Days I Just Want To Lie Down And Die

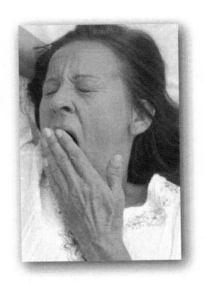

"I am so tired, my tired is tired"

L. B.

If I were to ask you about the menopause symptom that troubles you the most, you may say hot flashes or mood swings or disturbed sleep or joint pain. You may say that it is a combination of some, or many, of the 30 or more menopause symptoms.

However when I ask women to tell me the worst thing about menopause, the most common answers are:

1. I feel tired all the time.
2. I am exhausted.
3. I have no energy.

If you are fatigued all the time and/or have no energy, it will be caused by one or more of the following conditions, which are rife during menopause:

- Sleep deprivation – many women have trouble falling asleep or staying asleep, or a combination of both, during menopause.
- Stress – it may keep you awake … but even if it doesn't, stress in itself is draining. It saps energy and tires.
- Hypothyroidism (underactive thyroid).
- Insulin resistance.
- Adrenal fatigue.
- Crashing fatigue syndrome.

While each of these conditions may have its own cause and treatment/ remedy to relieve it, there is a common denominator associated them.

Hormonal imbalance is the common denominator cause of fatigue during menopause. Your body operates as a holistic system. It is like an orchestra. The various parts of your body are like the musicians and your hormones are like the conductor of the orchestra.

Hormones are chemical messengers that direct your body to perform specific tasks. A balanced hormonal state is essential to all functions in your body.

Prior to perimenopause, your hormones work in harmony by co-existing with one another in a certain ratio. This keeps your body healthy and functioning.

During perimenopause, your ovaries produce less estrogen and progesterone. While estrogen levels fall from their premenopausal levels during perimenopause, progesterone levels fall further. In terms of the ratio between them, there is greater percentage of estrogen in your body, relative to progesterone (1).

The change in the ratio between estrogen and progesterone disturbs the balance between all the hormones in your body. This affects the functioning of all of the systems of your body.

In essence here is what happens:

1. The ratio between estrogen and progesterone in your body is disturbed during menopause. This brings about the various physical, mental and emotional symptoms of menopause.
2. The physical, mental and emotional symptoms cause ongoing stress, prompting your adrenal glands to produce increasing amounts of cortisol.
3. High levels of cortisol slow down production of thyroid hormone, which leads to hypothyroidism.
4. Hypothyroidism leads to decreased insulin sensitivity (the body is not using insulin correctly to provide the cells of the body with the energy they need). The body increases its production of insulin to try to give the cells of the body the energy it needs, but fails.
5. Hypothyroidism and decreased insulin sensitivity increases stress on the body on an ongoing basis. This causes cortisol levels to be permanently high. The adrenal glands begin to produce decreasing amounts of cortisol. They are unable to meet the demand for cortisol. The adrenal glands become exhausted.
6. Your body doesn't just use cortisol to deal with stressful situations. Optimal cortisol levels are needed for your thyroid (2) to function as it should. In the face of insufficient cortisol, your thyroid starts

to work overtime to produce more thyroid hormones. This leads to thyroid exhaustion. Your body produces insufficient thyroid hormones (under-active thyroid).

7.   Hormonal imbalance interferes with sleep. An imbalance in one hormone causes an imbalance in other hormones, and so on. ....The cycle of hormonal imbalance perpetuates itself.

The end result is that you feel wiped out – exhausted and without energy.

HOW TO RELIEVE FATIGUE, EXHAUSTION AND LACK OF ENERGY?

If fatigue, exhaustion and lack of energy are caused by hormonal imbalance, doesn't it make sense to you that if you re-balance your hormones you will relieve these symptoms.

There is only one way in which you can re-balance your hormones: have a test to determine the level of your hormones and consult with a hormone expert to re-balance them based on the results of the test.

This is a form of hormone therapy (HT). It is called bio-identical hormone therapy. This method is very different than the conventional hormone therapy recommended by most doctors.

Conventional HT does not involve testing your hormone levels. It involves a prescription that will increase the level of estrogen in your body, regardless of the levels of any of the other hormones in your body. It is based on the supposition that as estrogen levels fall during menopause, that this is the cause of menopause symptoms .... And that if estrogen is increased menopause symptoms will be relieved.

It is true that estrogen levels fall during menopause, but it is not true that falling estrogen levels is the cause of your menopause symptoms. The cause of your menopause symptoms is too much estrogen in your body, relative to progesterone, which triggers changes in the levels of all the other hormones. More estrogen is the last thing that you need!

As many women are averse to hormone therapy of any kind, I will discuss the above conditions that cause exhaustion, fatigue and lack of energy in subsequent posts and non- hormonal treatments and remedies that may help to relieve them.

2

Do You Feel Tire All the Time?

"Fatigue is an excellent gauge of well-being because it is a very hard symptom to mask..."

KATHLEEN A. KENDALL-TACKETT

There can be no doubt that the symptoms of menopause can cause disturbed sleep that result in severe fatigue.

However, did you know that extreme tiredness is not just experienced by menopausal women? Dr. John Tintera, an endocrinologist, found that up to 67% of the general population experiences symptoms of fatigue (3) and that 16% are severe sufferers.

Therefore if you feel tired all the time, the cause of it may not just be menopause symptoms. What else may be causing your tiredness?

26% of menopausal women have an under-active thyroid condition (4). This causes them to feel tired all the time. Many other menopausal woman have adrenal fatigue....and don't know it. They just assume that their fatigue is caused by menopause.

WHAT IS ADRENAL FATIGUE?

Your adrenal glands, the tiny thumb-shaped glands that sit over your kidneys, are responsible for regulating your body's response to stress by controlling the hormones released during stress.

When these glands are functioning optimally, they produce three hormones that help you to deal with stressful circumstances....cortisol, epinephrine (also called adrenaline) and DHEA. Cortisol is the primary stress hormone. It may be helpful to think of your adrenal glands as your primary shock absorbers.

If your stress becomes chronic, or is not well managed, your adrenal glands are unable to function optimally. When you are consistently under stress, your adrenal glands are working overtime to produce the hormones necessary to help you deal with the stress.

Eventually, they run out of steam, and stop producing sufficient hormones. Adrenal fatigue (5) occurs when your adrenal glands cannot adequately meet the demands of stress.

Menopause is a time of increased stress.....both physical stress and emotional stress. When a menopausal woman experiences adrenal fatigue, menopause has likely played a significant role in bringing it on.

HOW TO TELL IF YOU HAVE ADRENAL FATIGUE?

The dominating symptom is fatigue – a fatigue that cannot be relieved by prolonged rest.

James Wilson, PhD, the author of the book Adrenal Fatigue, writes that adrenal fatigue symptoms include (6):

- Trouble getting out of bed in the morning.
- Chronic tiredness, even after you wake up in the morning.
- Trouble thinking clearly or finishing your tasks.

Another sign of adrenal fatigue is a craving for salty and sweet snacks.

HOW ESTROGEN AND PROGESTERONE LEVELS ARE LINKED TO ADRENAL FATIGUE?

Your body operates as a holistic system. It is like an orchestra. The various parts of your body are like the musicians and your hormones are like the conductor of the orchestra. Hormones are chemical messengers that direct your body to perform specific tasks. A balanced hormonal state is essential to all functions in your body.

Prior to perimenopause, your hormones work in harmony by co-existing with one another in a certain ratio. Your hormones are said to be balanced. This keeps your body healthy and functioning.

During perimenopause, the pattern of estrogen levels changes. Estrogen levels are higher than they were prior to the onset of perimenopause (7). While estrogen levels are generally higher during perimenopause, the levels fluctuate. They surge and dip cyclically. Progesterone levels fall consistently during perimenopause.

In terms of the ratio between them, there is greater percentage of estrogen in your body, relative to progesterone. This creates a condition called estrogen dominance.

Estrogen dominance is the trigger that causes all menopause symptoms. As estrogen dominance affects all of the hormones in your body and your hormones control all of the functions of your body, it is also the cause of a under-active thyroid condition, insulin intolerance, adrenal fatigue and many other conditions that can leave you feeling tired all the time

Your cortisol levels are affected by this. Progesterone is a precursor hormone to cortisol. A precursor hormone is a hormone that makes another hormone, especially by metabolic reaction.

In essence here is what happens that causes adrenal fatigue and leaves you feeling tired all the time:

1. Estrogen dominance causes your menopause symptoms.
2. When your menopause symptoms are moderate to severe, they cause increasing physical and emotional stress.
3. When you experience stress, your body produces increasing amounts of cortisol to deal with the stress.
4. Chronic stress demands more cortisol than your body is able to produce, because progesterone levels are falling during perimenopause and low after menopause.

WHAT TO DO IF YOU FEEL TIRED ALL THE TIME?

The first thing you should do is see your doctor to ensure that there isn't a serious health condition that is causing your exhaustion.

Assuming that your doctor does not find a serious health condition, the most effective way to treat feeling tired all the time is to get the levels of your hormones tested and then re-balanced. This will correct estrogen dominance and eliminate most, if not all, of your menopause symptoms.

However this is a costly option and may be beyond the financial means of many women. There will be lab fees (hundreds of dollars) to test your hormone levels and physician fees to help you re-balance them. Often, this is not covered by health insurance policies.

A safe, effective and inexpensive way to relieve your symptoms is to use progesterone therapy – self- administered natural progesterone cream. Natural progesterone cream will increase your progesterone level and reduce your estrogen levels (8).

Another effective treatment for disturbed sleep during menopause is Cognitive Behavioral Therapy (CBT). Controlled medical trials have found that CBT effectively relieves insomnia (9).

CBT trains people to use techniques that address the mental (or cognitive) factors associated with insomnia, such as the 'racing mind', and to overcome the worry and other negative emotions that accompany the experience of being unable to sleep. Medical trials have also found that CBT relieves hot flashes and night sweats.

3

Tired When You Get Up .... And Tired Throughout The Day?

*"I'd give anything for a good night's sleep I am tired all day long.
I go to bed tired, but I have trouble falling asleep. When I finally
do fall asleep, I have trouble staying asleep. How I miss the days
when I could sleep 9-12 hours like dead!"*

L. G.

Sounds familiar?

If your head and your pillow are not spending much quality time together, you are not alone. 61% of women experience menopause insomnia, according to the National Sleep Foundation (10). To put this into perspective for you, it is estimated that there are 50 million American women who are currently experiencing menopause symptoms. That means that there are approximately 30 million American women, who are experiencing disturbed sleep during menopause.

A recent sleep survey (11) revealed that 63 percent of menopausal women struggle to fall asleep and 79 percent have trouble staying asleep.

THE CAUSE OF DISTURBED SLEEP DURING MENOPAUSE:

Your body operates as a holistic system. It is like an orchestra. The various parts of your body are like the musicians and your hormones are like the conductor of the orchestra. Hormones are chemical messengers that direct your body to perform specific tasks. A balanced hormonal state is essential to all functions in your body.

Prior to perimenopause, your hormones worked in harmony by co-existing with one another in a certain ratio. This kept your body healthy and functioning.

During perimenopause, your ovaries produce less estrogen and progesterone than they did prior to perimenopause. While estrogen levels fall from their pre-premenopausal levels during perimenopause, progesterone levels fall further. In terms of the ratio between them, there is greater percentage of estrogen in your body, relative to progesterone. There is an imbalance between them, when compared to their pre-perimenopause levels.

In post menopause your body produces zero progesterone, but it continues to produce a little estrogen. This perpetuates the imbalance between estrogen and progesterone.

The change in the ratio between estrogen and progesterone disturbs the balance between all the hormones in your body. This triggers changes in the levels of all the hormones in your body, which is the cause of all of your menopause symptoms.

WHICH HORMONAL CHANGES ARE MOST RESPONSIBLE FOR DISTURBED SLEEP DURING MENOPAUSE?

The hormones that have the biggest impact on menopause insomnia are

- Estrogen
- Progesterone
- Cortisol

Estrogen encourages wakefulness. It has an arousal effect (12), which makes it more difficult to sleep. Falling estrogen levels causes hot flashes and night sweats and interferes with sleep.

Progesterone has a sedative affect (13). It makes you feel drowsy. It shares a close relationship with GABA, a neuro-chemical in your brain that calms your nervous system. This has the effect of reducing those clamoring thoughts chasing round your head so you can relax and drift off to sleep more easily.

During perimenopause there is more estrogen relative to progesterone, when compared to their levels prior to perimenopause. In post menopause there is no progesterone, but a little estrogen. The change in the ratio between them affects sleep for the obvious reason — there is too much of the estrogen arousal effect compared to the calming progesterone effect. As a result, the brain can't calm down enough to rest.

Cortisol is the stress hormone. It prepares your body to meet real and imagined threats, stress. Your body increases production of cortisol when you feel stress.

During menopause, its symptoms cause mental, emotional, and physical stress. When the symptoms are moderate to severe, the level of cortisol can be permanently raised.

Anxiety, mood swings and depression (14) are some of the common symptoms of menopause that are associated with higher levels of cortisol. If any of these symptoms are present when you lay your body down to sleep, your cortisol levels will be high. Your body will be in a "high alert" state, prepared to deal with a threat. This is not conducive to falling asleep.

On the other side of the coin, if you have been experiencing sleep disturbance for an extended period of time, you will be exhausted. This in itself will increase your stress levels… and cortisol level. You lay your weary body down to sleep, but you are anxious about not being able to fall asleep … because of all of the previous nights when you were unable to fall asleep. And so the cycle, as well as your sleep disturbance, perpetuates itself.

HOW TO RELIEVE DISTURBED SLEEP DURING MENOPAUSE AND POST MENOPAUSE?

As disturbed sleep during menopause is caused by hormonal imbalance, if you re-balance your hormones your sleep will normalize. This involves taking bioidentical hormones.

Many women are averse to hormone therapy of any kind.

Another effective treatment for disturbed sleep during menopause is Cognitive Behavioral Therapy (CBT). Controlled medical trials have found that CBT effectively relieves insomnia.

CBT trains people to use techniques that address the mental (or cognitive) factors associated with insomnia, such as the 'racing mind', and to overcome the worry and other negative emotions that accompany the experience of being unable to sleep. Medical trials have also found that CBT relieves hot flashes and night sweats.

CBT is of particular interest because another factor that affects sleep is aging. A Sleep Foundation study (16) has found that as women age, increasing numbers of women encounter sleep difficulties. The majority of postmenopausal women experience sleep disturbance. A lower percentage of premenopausal woman suffer from insomnia. An even smaller percentage of pre-premenopausal women encounter sleep disturbance.

4

You Need To Re-Think Your Strategy For Dealing With Hot Flashes

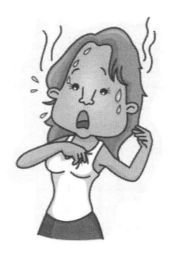

"How much longer will I have to suffer?"

G. L.

Conventional wisdom has it that hot flashes will last for just a few years. The treatment recommended by doctors to relieve them, Traditional HRT, is based on the assumption that they will last for just a few years.

Yet a new study (16) of 1,449 menopausal women has found the following:

- Hot flashes last for 7.4 years on average. Half of the women in the study experienced them for less than that time, but half experienced them for more than that time ... some for as long as 14 years.
- Women who started experiencing them when they were still having regular periods (12% of the women) experienced them for an average of 11.8 years.
- Women who first experience them after their periods had permanently stopped (20% of the women), experienced them for the shortest amount of time, an average of 3.4 years.
- 65% of the women started to experience them when their periods became irregular.
- After menopause (no more periods), they lasted for 4.5 years on average.

The message is clear: hot flashes last for a longer period of time than you and the doctors may have expected.

CONSEQUENCES FOR WOMEN TAKING TRADITIONAL HRT:

The treatment for hot flashes that is recommended by most doctors is traditional HRT. It is effective in relieving them. However, many medical studies have found that traditional HRT increases the user's risk of breast cancer, heart disease and stroke.

For this reason, doctors advise that traditional HRT should be taken for just a short period of time to minimize the health risks. Short period of time is not defined, but most doctors take it to mean no more than 3-5 years.

However the new hot flash study has revealed that most menopausal women experience hot flashes for longer than that.

What can a woman do if she is experiencing moderate to severe hot flashes?

You may do the following:

1. Take traditional HRT for as long as you experience them. If your they last for longer than 3-5 years, your health risks will increase but your quality of life will be better
2. Take traditional HRT for no longer than 3-5 years and then stop.

However, a study of 8,400 postmenopausal women (17) found that more than half of the women, who started taking traditional HRT to relieve hot flashes and other symptoms, saw a dramatic resurgence of those symptoms when they discontinued the therapy.

When you stop taking traditional HRT, you will need to find another alternative to deal with your hot flashes

3. An increasing number of women are turning to bioidentical hormone therapy for hot flash relief and relief of other menopause symptoms. It provides effective hot flash relief.

Medical studies have not found any health risks associated with taking it. Therefore you can take it for as long as hot flashes persist.

4. Many women seek and find hot flash relief from non-hormonal treatments and remedies such as:

> Weight loss – Overweight women, who lost weight, experienced a significant hot flash reduction.

> Diet – hot flash frequency is suppressed after eating, while hot flashes are experienced when blood glucose falls between meals. Maintaining stability in blood glucose level may be effective in reducing menopausal hot flashes.

Exercise– Results are inconclusive. However, aerobic exercise as part of a weight loss program for overweight menopausal women is effective at hot flash reduction.

Soy – this study says that it is effective. Other studies raise a question about its effectiveness.

Black Cohosh – It's widely used, but some research questions its effectiveness. In a year-long clinical trial funded by the US National Institutes of Health, it was found to be no better than a placebo for relieving hot flashes.

Pycnogenol – Found to be very effective (18).

Hypnosis – clinical hypnosis results in significant hot flash reductions.

Relaxation Therapy – Significant hot flash reductions.

Acupuncture – Significant hot flash reductions.

Yoga – A 30% hot flash reduction.

Deep Breathing – results in a hot flash reduction.

Bio identical hormone therapy – There have been no independent studies conducted on its effectiveness for hot flash relief. However many women say that they have benefited from it.

Each of these treatments and remedies has helped some women. None of them have helped all women!

It is worth pursuing this option to see if you can find a treatment or remedy that works for you.

5. A proven way to reduce the frequency and severity of your hot flashes is to reduce the level of stress you are experiencing.

A study (19) was conducted to determine the effect that stress has on hot flashes. The researchers found that:

- Women who rated themselves as "moderately anxious", due to life stresses, experienced three times as many hot flashes compared with women who were within "normal" anxiety range.
- Women with "high" anxiety scores experienced five times as many hot flashes.

Women who experience moderate to severe hot flashes say that menopause is the most stressful phase of their lives. If you increase your understanding of stress and how to reduce it, you can reduce their frequency and severity.

WHAT IS STRESS?
Stress is difficult to define because it is subjective. What causes you to feel stress during menopause may not cause another woman to feel stress … and vice versa. Having said that, here is a definition of stress that I favor:

Stress is a feeling of anxiety and tension brought about by anything that you perceive to be a threat to your well-being. It is a physiological, mental and emotional reaction to that threat.

The most important word in the above definition is "perceive". The definition of perceive is *to interpret or regard someone or something in a particular way.*

If you experience severe and/or frequent menopause symptoms, you probably perceive them as a threat to your well-being. Per the definition of stress above, they will be a stressful experience for you … for as long as you regard them in that way.

Stress has a close cousin. It is anxiety. Anxiety is defined as a feeling of worry, nervousness, or unease about something with an uncertain outcome.

Stress and anxiety go hand in hand. Anxiety is most commonly triggered by the stress in our lives.

What is the difference between stress and anxiety? Stress is a reaction to something happening now. Anxiety is a reaction to something that is going to happen at a future date, may happen at a future date, or may never actually happen at all.

Some ways to reduce stress during menopause (or at any time):

- Any type of meditation will reduce stress (20). Meditation is a practice of concentrated focus upon a sound, object, visualization, the breath etc. for an extended period of time. In so doing, your breathing slows down and your stress level falls.
- Yoga will reduce stress. In yoga, the body, breath and mind are seen as key aspects of each and every human being. The system, and various techniques of yoga, increases tranquility and clarity of the mind.
- Relaxation therapy reduces stress. It is a technique involving breathing therapy, which focuses on helping you relax each of your muscle groups and therefore achieving overall relaxation. You are shown how to do the technique so you can continue the therapy at home.
- Music has the power to improve mood and reduce stress during menopause. Listening to music that you love, and that fits whatever mood you're in, has been shown to lower stress levels (21).
- Having fun and laughing reduces stress levels. Try to find ways in your daily life to have fun, laugh and joke as much as possible and you'll lower your stress level during menopause.

- Increase your intake of vitamin B6, vitamin B5 (pantothenic acid), and vitamin C. These nutrients play an important role in your body's regulation of cortisol (the stress hormone) levels. The levels of these nutrients are depleted by stress.

Additionally, if you eat right and exercise every day, it will help you to reduce stress during menopause.

5

Say Goodbye to Hot Flashes ... Without Taking Hormones or Drugs

"The first indication of menopause is a broken thermo-stat.....God; middle age is an unending insult."

DOROTHEA BENTON FRANK

Suppose there is a safe and effective treatment for hot flashes that you don't know about, which is recommended by the following:

- The North American Menopause Society (NAMS)
- The American Cancer Society
- Breast Cancer.Org
- Other prestigious medical bodies
- Major woman's health organizations

My guess is that you would want to know about it. Some of you may also want to know why you haven't heard of it already. The treatment is called CBT – Cognitive Behavioral Therapy.

WHAT IS CBT?
It is a therapy that trains people to use techniques that helps them control and even prevent their symptoms.

CBT can be done in 3 ways:

1. Working 1:1 with a therapist.
2. As part of a group.
3. By yourself, using self-help (booklet and CD).

CBT Effectively provides relief from hot flashes.

Medical trials (22) have found that CBT provides effective relief from hot flashes and night sweats, as well as depression, anxiety, mood swings and insomnia. It helps women deal with stress caused by menopause, which exacerbates symptoms.

The trials found that all 3 methods of CBT effectively reduce hot flashes and night sweats. Each of the methods improved quality of life as well.

The North American Menopause Society (NAMS) reported that the studies found that CBT achieved a reduction in frequency and severity associated with hot flashes, depression, anxiety, and an overall improvement in quality of life. They said that CBT was found to be effective for healthy premenopausal and postmenopausal women, as well as women with menopausal symptoms induced or exacerbated by breast cancer treatments. (23)

The American Cancer Society said:

"After breast cancer treatment, 65% to 85% of women experience hot flashes and night sweats – many of them severe enough to affect sleep, mood, and quality of life. These symptoms are challenging to treat because the most effective therapy, hormone treatment with estrogen and progesterone, can increase chances of the cancer returning and is therefore not often an option for breast cancer survivors. A new study by British researchers found that cognitive behavioral therapy (CBT) can help women safely manage their hot flashes and night sweats".(24)

BreastCancer.org reported that besides less severe hot flashes, women who got cognitive therapy were more likely to report better overall health, better emotional health, fewer sleep problems, and better memory and concentration. (25)

So, why you haven't heard about CBT for hot flashes before now?

Chances are your doctor has not spoken to you about CBT for your hot flashes. Your doctor may not even know that medical trials have verified the effectiveness of CBT in connection with relieving hot flash torment.

Doctors receive their information about menopause treatments directly from pharmaceutical companies and medical journals that are promoting the conventional medical treatments- drugs. They do not promote the benefits of CBT for the relief of menopause symptoms.

6

Hot Flash Relief ...S-Equol Nutritional Supplement Is Effective

"I expected this to stop, or at least decrease, by now"

M. A.

Dr Wulf H. Utian, M.D., Ph.D., D.Sc. Founder of the North American Menopause Society (NAMS) and Director Emeritus of the Department of Obstetrics and Gynecology, University Hospitals of Cleveland has said this about S-equol:

"Current data suggest that women may have benefits with S-equol for meno-pausal vasomotor symptoms (hot flashes and night sweats) and possibly additional benefits, such as skin health. Given the studies supporting safety of S-equol, physi-cians and health care professionals may consider the use of S-equol as a future first round option for menopause symptoms, especially for women not wanting to use pharmaceuticals".

Controlled clinical studies have documented that a supplement containing S-equol is safe and effective for hot flash relief...in post-menopausal wom-en. It has also been found to effectively relieve postmenopausal muscle and joint pain. (26)

Equol comes from soy. When soy is eaten certain bacteria in the gut change chemicals contained in soy to equol. However, only 30-60% of people are able to break down soy chemicals to form equol. Some studies have shown that people capable of breaking soy down to form equol get more health benefits from soy. These people are called "equol producers."

S-equol is a natural supplement. It mimics some, but not all, activities of estrogen. It has many of the positive qualities of estrogen, without its potentially harmful effects.

HRT, which is primarily estrogen hormone therapy, increases a woman's estrogen levels. It is effective in the relief of hot flashes, but it increases a women's risk of breast cancer, heart disease and stroke.

S-equol effectively relieves hot flashes, without increasing your health risks.

How S-equol relieves post menopause hot flashes and night sweats

Hot flashes and night sweats are associated with low levels of estrogen in post menopause.

During perimenopause estrogen levels are falling from their pre-perimenopause levels. In post menopause, estrogen levels bottom out and stay low. About 6 months before menopause (12 consecutive months without a period), estrogen levels drop significantly. (27) Estrogen levels bottom out during post menopause, but not to zero. While your ovaries no longer produce estrogen, your body makes estrogen in other ways.

Hot flashes tend to intensify during post menopause. According to the National Institute of Health (NIH) (28), the percentage of women experiencing them increases sharply in the 2 years before final menstrual period and peaks 1 year after final menstrual period.

Experts don't know exactly why this happens, but it's believed to be related to the hypothalamus, the portion of the brain that regulates temperature. The hypothalamus is acutely sensitive to estrogen levels.

In 2014 a study (29) that followed 255 women for 16 years – from pre-menopause to post menopause – reported its findings. It found that moderate to severe hot flashes continue, on average, for nearly 5 years during post menopause and that more than one third of women experienced them for 10 years or more during post menopause.

Therefore, hot flash relief is a subject of great interest to many postmenopausal women.

Taking S-equol supplements has the same effect in your body as raising the level of estrogen by taking HRT, without increasing your health risks.

Do not take S-equol for hot flash relief during perimenopause!

Contrary to what you may have been led to believe, perimenopause symptoms are not caused by decreasing estrogen levels. Extensive medical research has revealed that estrogen levels are higher during perimenopause than they are in younger women. (30)

Dr Steven R. Goldstein, MD, professor of obstetrics and gynecology at New York University's Langone Medical Center says: *"It's the paradox of perimenopause. Estrogen levels go up before they go down".*

While estrogen levels are in a higher range during perimenopause, than they are prior to perimenopause, they are fluctuating. This means that their levels go up and down. They surge and fall cyclically.

Progesterone levels are consistently falling throughout perimenopause. This coupled with the higher levels of estrogen creates the condition known as estrogen dominance.

If you take S-equol supplements during perimenopause, it will have the effect of raising estrogen levels even higher, which will worsen your hot flashes. In fact, the most effective way to relieve hot flashes during perimenopause is to increase your progesterone level.

7

Breaking News...How Long Will Your Hot Flashes Last?

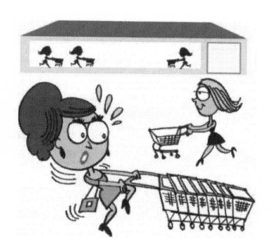

"Hot flashes are driving me crazy"

M.B.

Hot flashes affect approximately 80% of menopausal woman. Women typically expect them to persist for just a few years.

A new study (31) has found that hot flashes can continue for as long as 14 years and the earlier they begin the longer a woman is likely to experience them.

The study found that women who experience hot flashes in early peri-menopause can expect to experience them for more years than women who first experience them later in the menopause passage.

The researchers followed 1,449 women, who had frequent hot flashes and night sweats, for 17 years. None of the women used hormone replacement treatments. None of the women in the study had a hysterectomy. All of the women had their ovaries intact.

A summary of the findings of the study:

- Women whose hot flashes started after their periods stopped experienced hot flashes for a total of 3.4 years … on average. This accounted for a small minority of the women …. Approximately 20%.
- Women who started getting hot flashes when they were still having regular periods, or were in early perimenopause, experienced hot flashes and night sweats for a total of 11.8 years … on average. On average, they experienced hot flashes and night sweats for approximately 9 years after their periods stopped.
- The overall average length of time the 1,449 women experienced hot flashes and night sweats was 7.4 years.
- Half of the women experienced hot flashes and night sweats for longer than 7.4 years — some of these women had them for 14 years.

RELEVANT FINDINGS FROM OTHER HOT FLASH STUDIES:

In 2014 a study (32) that followed 255 women for 16 years – from pre-menopause to post menopause – reported its findings. It found that moderate to severe hot flashes continue, on average, for nearly 5 years during post menopause and that more than one third of women experienced moderate to severe hot flashes for 10 years or more during post menopause.

An earlier study (33) that followed 436 menopausal women from 1995 – 2009 (thirteen years) shed more light on post menopause hot flashes. All of the women were between the ages of 35-47 in 1995.

Earlier, I mentioned STRAW system and its stages of menopause. As a reminder, Perimenopause consists of two stages – early menopause transition and late menopause transition. Post menopause consists of 2 stages – early post menopause and late post menopause.

The STRAW reminder would help to understand the findings of the 436 women study:

- The median duration of moderate to severe hot flashes was 10.2 years.
- Women whose moderate to severe hot flashes commenced in the early menopause transition stage had a median duration of 7.35 years.
- Women whose moderate to severe hot flashes commenced in the late menopause transition to early post menopause stage had a median duration of 3.84 years.
- The most common ages at onset of moderate to severe hot flashes were 45–49 years. For this group, the median duration was 8.1 years.

One more pertinent fact about hot flashes ….. According to the National Institute of Health (NIH) (33), the percentage of women experiencing hot flashes increases sharply in the two years before final menstrual period and peaks one year after final menstrual period.

WHAT THE FINDINGS OF THESE STUDIES MEANS TO YOU?

Chances are that if you are reading this post, you are experiencing moderate to severe hot flashes. If they were mild you probably wouldn't bother reading this post.

What probably interests you most is to learn how long they may last and how to relieve/reduce them. Hopefully, the information provided in this post thus far has improved your understanding about duration of hot flashes. In terms of hot flash relief, you can either use hormonal treatments or non-hormonal treatments and remedies.

An array of non-hormonal remedies and treatments exists ... from taking various herbs to treatments like acupuncture ... that have relieved hot flashes for many women.

Doctors most often recommend hormone replacement therapy (conventional HRT) to relieve hot flashes. Conventional HRT increases the level of estradiol (1 of the 3 estrogens in a woman's body) in your body. Studies show that it is effective at relieving hot flashes, but it increases the risk of breast cancer and stroke when it is taken.

Because of the health risks associated with taking conventional HRT, doctors say it should be taken for the shortest time possible. Some medical authorities have advised that it should be taken for no more than 2-3 years. The consensus seems to be to take it for no more than 5 years.

Using conventional HRT to relieve hot flashes is a problematical solution because a majority of women experience hot flashes for more than 5 years, per the findings of the hot flash studies. Therefore a woman can either continue to take conventional HRT after 5 years, in which case her health risks increase or she can stop taking it. If she stops taking it, the hot flashes will return.

A study (34) of 8,400 menopausal women, who started taking hormone therapy to relieve hot flashes, saw a dramatic resurgence of hot flashes when they discontinued the therapy. Another study found that women, who had been on hormone therapy and stopped, experienced more hot flashes than women who had never been on it.

An effective alternative to conventional HRT for hot flash relief is bio-identical hormone therapy. It entails testing to determine the hormone levels in your body and then re-balancing the levels of your hormones, using natural hormones that do the identical things in your body as the hormones produced by your body. The bio-identical estrogen used is not estradiol. It is estriol, which is weakest of the 3 estrogens.

There is no known health risks associated with taking bio-identical hormones. Therefore bio-identical hormones can be used for as long as you experience hot flashes.

8

I've Known Her Forever .... But Her Name Escapes Me

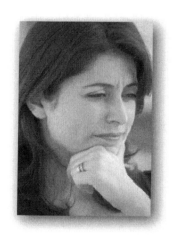

"I feel like I am losing my mind"

J.L.

J ean took a seat in my office. She looked perturbed. Then she blurted out:

"I was standing in front of the yogurt shop the other day with my mom and my sister when a friend approached. We exchanged hugs and I attempted to make introductions.

"This is my mom Mary and my sister Barbara." When it came time to iden-tify my friend, I drew a blank. So I said, "This is my dear friend who takes great, great care of me." I hugged her again to distract from the omission.

My mind flashed on: "her daughter ice skates, she has one of those tiny little dogs, she's a poet. Dang, what is her name?" It didn't come to me. Until five minutes later."

She said that this sort of thing was happening to her increasingly. It was embarrassing her and upsetting her.

She said that she is aware that it happens to many menopausal women, but that knowing that does not allay her fear that she is losing her mind. She wanted to know if there was something she could do about it.

Jean's menopause brain fog experience is more than common. Research reveals that up to two thirds of women experience menopause brain fog. Brain fog can be described as feelings of mental confusion or lack of mental clarity. It is called brain fog because it can feel like a cloud that reduces your ability to think clearly.

Here are some common brain fog experiences:

- Brain freeze – difficulty recalling words, names, addresses, phone numbers etc., which you know very well. Very often it feels like the information is "just out of reach" or "on the tip of my tongue".
- Memory lapses – difficulty recalling recent events.
- Forgetfulness – can't remember where you left something …. Could be a car, phone, glasses, keys etc.
- Impaired concentration – thoughts wander a great deal making it difficult to do a task. This makes learning difficult as well.

THE CAUSE OF MENOPAUSE BRAIN FOG:

First let me say that it is a misnomer to call it menopause brain fog. Brain fog is most common during perimenopause. It is relatively uncommon af-ter menopause (when a woman experiences her final menstrual period).

You may attribute your menopause brain fog, like your other perimenopause symptoms, to the changing levels of estrogen and progesterone in your body, and in a sense this is true. During perimenopause, there is a greater percentage of estrogen in your body, relative to progesterone, than prior to perimenopause. This condition is known as estrogen dominance.

Estrogen dominance triggers changes in the levels of the rest of the hormones in your body. It also triggers changes in chemicals in your brain, called neurotransmitters.

There are ten billion neurons (brain cells) in your brain. Between each of these neurons are neurotransmitters. (35) Neurotransmitters are chemical messengers that transmit thought from one cell to the next, allowing your brain cells to "talk to each other".

Neurotransmitters control all of your mental and emotional responses.

The relationship between hormones and your neurotransmitters can best be described as one of master and servant. Your hormones send messages to your body, instructing it to do certain functions. Your neurotransmitters carry those messages to your body.

The changes in the levels of estrogen and progesterone, and the ratios between them, trigger a chain reaction of change in the levels of your neurotransmitters. It is actually the changing levels of your neurotransmitters that cause the brain fog.

Also, there is a nutrient that has significant effects on your brain function. It is vitamin D.

Vitamin D deficiency is associated with these menopause brain fog symptoms.

Your vitamin D level affects the neurotransmitter system in your brain.

One study has found that people with vitamin D deficiency performed poorly on cognitive tests. The researchers concluded that that there is an association between low vitamin D status and cognitive impairment. (36)

Researchers have found that vitamin D improves brain function, aids in neurotransmitter synthesis, promotes nerve growth, improves your memory, increases awareness, regulates your moods, removes toxins from your body that can cause brain fog and transports oxygen, blood and nutrients to your brain.

The neurotransmitters epinephrine and norepinephrine are closely linked to menopause brain fog symptoms. They regulate attention, mental focus, memory, learning and cognition.

Low levels of vitamin D bring about low levels of epinephrine and norepinephrine and therefor menopause brain fog symptoms.

There is also a strong link between vitamin D deficiency and Alzheimer Disease. (36)

It is important to get your vitamin D level tested.

HOW TO RELIEVE MENOPAUSE BRAIN FOG?

1. Get your vitamin D level tested. (37) If the test reveals a deficiency, increase your intake of Vitamin D with via food/Vitamin D supplement.
2. Re-balance your levels of progesterone and estrogen.

The most effective way to do this is to first get the levels of your hormones tested and then re-balance them.

However this is a costly option and may be beyond the financial means of many women. There will be lab fees (hundreds of dollars) to test your hormone levels and physician fees to help you re-balance them. Often, this is not covered by health insurance policies.

A safe, effective and inexpensive way to re-balance your hormones is to use progesterone therapy – self-administered natural progesterone cream. Natural progesterone cream will increase your progesterone level and help to regulate your estrogen levels.

9

Menopause Brain Fog – You Don't Have To Be Embarrassed Anymore

Is this the onset of dementia?

Does menopause brain fog make you feel stupid?

Are you embarrassed in a social or work setting when you can't remember the name of someone you know very well, or you cannot recall a common word, when you are mid-sentence?

Does it frustrate you when you speak gibberish during a conversation?

Do you walk into a room, and can't remember why you went there?

Are you forever misplacing things like your keys, phone or even your car?

Do you worry that brain fog will be with you permanently?

Right now there are more than 30 million menopausal women in the US alone ... just like you ... who are experiencing memory loss, confusion, lack of concentration and a general decrease in their cognitive abilities – the symptoms of menopause brain fog.

There is no way of telling how many more women are experiencing this worldwide. Perhaps it is in the hundreds of millions, as research has revealed that 2 out of 3 women experience menopause brain fog ... to some degree.

Does it comfort you to know that you share brain fog with so many other women? Probably not. However it may comfort you to know that you don't have to experience these symptoms any longer.

During perimenopause, the ratio of estrogen to progesterone significantly changes.

Contrary to what you may have been led to believe, menopause brain fog and the other symptoms experienced during perimenopause are not caused by low estrogen levels. Extensive medical research has revealed that estrogen levels are higher during perimenopause than they are in younger women. (38)

Dr Steven R. Goldstein, MD, (39) professor of obstetrics and gynecology at New York University's Langone Medical Center says:

> *"It's the paradox of perimenopause. Estrogen levels go up before they go down."*

While estrogen levels are in a higher range during perimenopause, than they are prior to perimenopause, they are fluctuating. This means that their levels go up and down. They surge and fall cyclically, while the level of progesterone falls consistently.

As a result, there is a greater percentage of estrogen in your body, relative to progesterone. This is known as the estrogen dominance.

Your body functions as a holistic system. Changes in one part of your body affects other parts of your body.

As mentioned in the previous chapter, while changes in the levels of estrogen and progesterone affect all of the other hormones in your body, they also affect the levels of the neurotransmitters in your brain.

The neurotransmitters are chemical messengers that transmit thought from one cell to the next, allowing your brain cells to "talk to each other".

There are 3 neurotransmitters that have a significant effect on how your brain functions. (40)

They are acetylcholine, serotonin, and norepinephrine. They have all been shown to regulate cognitive abilities. If there is a shortage in these neurotransmitters, there may be a decrease in cognitive function, leading to difficulty concentrating and memory lapses.

The levels of these neurotransmitters are affected by the levels of estrogen. When the levels of estrogen drop, as it does during one of its frequent fluctuations during perimenopause, the levels of these transmitters drop as well.

This makes perimenopause women susceptible to brain fog experiences.

In addition, estrogen helps regulate the level of blood flow to the brain. When levels of estrogen fall, blood flow to the brain decreases. This affects concentration and memory, as well.

Moreover, Low levels of progesterone were also directly contributes to poor memory and concentration difficulties. (41)

As prior discussed hormonal balance treatment, Vitamin D, and self-administered natural progesterone cream are in the cards to lift off that brain fog.

10

Vitamin D Deficiency, Menopause Brain Fog And Alzheimer's Disease

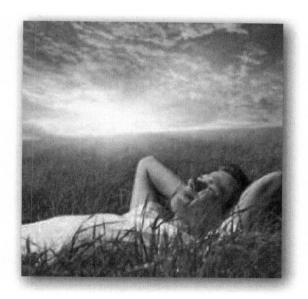

I s this the onset of Alzheimer's?

Imagine that there is a nutrient that could protect your brain. Imagine that if you have it in sufficient quantity that your menopause brain fog would be gone or greatly reduced.

This could mean no more of the following:

- Brain freeze
- Memory lapses
- Forgetfulness
- Impaired concentration
- Impaired thinking

There is a nutrient that has significant effects on your brain function. It is vitamin D. A Vitamin D deficiency brings about these menopause brain fog symptoms.

Vitamin D is called the "sunshine vitamin". It is unlike any other vitamin because it is produced by your body as a result of exposing your skin to the sun.

No other vitamin is produced by your body. They all come from the foods that you eat.

You wouldn't think that many women would be deficient in vitamin D, because all you have to do is to go outside in the sun for 15 minutes a day and your body will produce all of the vitamin D it needs.

However, more than 1 out of every 2 menopausal women is deficient in it. (42)

As mentioned before, Vitamin D deficiency is not the only cause of menopause brain fog. Falling levels of estrogen also causes it, but you can confuse the symptoms of vitamin D deficiency with the symptoms of menopause. They are very similar.

One study has found that people with vitamin D deficiency performed poorly on cognitive tests. The researchers concluded that that there is an association between low vitamin D status and cognitive impairment. (43)

Researchers have found that vitamin D improves brain function, aids in neurotransmitter synthesis, promotes nerve growth, improves your memory, increases awareness, regulates your moods, removes toxins from your body that can cause brain fog and transports oxygen, blood and nutrients to your brain.

Your vitamin D level affects the neurotransmitter system in your brain. When the levels of the neurotransmitters are altered, it affects your brain functions and causes menopause brain fog.

They regulate attention, mental focus, memory, learning and cognition. Low levels of vitamin D bring about low levels of epinephrine and norepinephrine and therefor menopause brain fog symptoms.

Not only does vitamin D deficiency cause menopause brain fog symptoms, but it significantly increases your risk of Alzheimer's disease and other types of dementia.

A recent study (44) evaluated vitamin D levels in 1658 people over 6 years. The researchers found that:

- People who were moderately deficient in vitamin D were 69% more likely to develop Alzheimer's disease than people with normal levels of vitamin D.
- People who were moderately deficient in vitamin D were 53% more likely to develop other forms of dementia than people with normal levels of vitamin D.
- People who were severely deficient in vitamin D were more than twice as likely to develop Alzheimer's disease, or another form of dementia, than people with normal levels of vitamin D.

Vitamin D deficiency has been found to significantly increase your risk of cancer, heart disease and other diseases – including diabetes, arthritis, osteoporosis and autoimmune diseases.

According to the Vitamin D Council, (45) there are 3 ways to test your Vitamin D level:

1. Ask your doctor for a vitamin D test. Be specific and ask for a 25(OH) D test. There is another type of blood test for vitamin D, called a 1,25(OH)$_2$D test, but the 25(OH)D test is the only one that will tell you whether you're getting enough vitamin D. If your health insurance covers a 25(OH) D test, this is a good way to work with your doctor to get tested.
2. Order an in-home test. These tests are sent to your home. You prick your finger and put a drop of blood on to some blotter paper. You send the paper to a laboratory to be tested. These are an alternative if you don't want to go to your doctor just for a vitamin D test, or if your insurance doesn't cover a test.
3. Order a test online and get blood work done at a laboratory. In the United States, there are a few websites that allow you to bypass your doctor and go straight to the testing laboratory. These websites include mymedlab.com, healthcheckusa.com and privatemdlabs.com. You can buy a 25(OH) D test from all of these companies and have the test itself done at your nearest LabCorp. These tests are a little more expensive than in-home tests.

Dr. JoAnn Manson, MD and past president of the North American Menopause Society (NAMS) said this about vitamin D: *"I think vitamin D is one of the most promising nutrients for prevention of cardiac disease and cancer, and I believe in it strongly." (46)*

Dr Manson is Professor of Medicine at Harvard Medical School, and Chief of Division of Preventive Medicine, Department of Medicine, at Brigham and Women's Hospital.

Dr Christiane Northrup, MD and bestselling author of "The Wisdom of Menopause" says that information about vitamin D can save your life.

11

Are Mood Swings Damaging Your Relationship With Family Or Friends?

"I'm what is known as premenopausal." "Peri", some of you may know, is a Latin prefix meaning 'SHUT YOUR FLIPPIN' __ __".

CELIA RIVENBARK

When I get bitchy...the bitch just comes out all on her own... like I've got no control over "HER".

This is what Helen said at the start of her appointment.

She explained she was feeling ok when she woke up. Then a little later...right out of the blue...she became angry, for no reason whatsoever. She said that the anger quickly turned to rage. When her husband asked her a perfectly innocent question, she flipped and screamed at him.

She said that prior to menopause she had always been a calm and laid back person and that she had not been her normal self since menopause.

She said that what was upsetting her the most was that her husband is such a good man and he had been particularly supportive of her, since the onset of her menopause.

She wanted to know what she could do to reduce her mood swings and manage them better.

To discuss the options available to her, it was necessary for her to have an understanding of the cause of mood swings during menopause. What follows is a synopsis of what we discussed for the remainder of her appointment.

Mood swings is a symptom experienced during perimenopause. Few women experience them after their final menstrual period. Therefore it would be more appropriate to refer to them as perimenopause mood swings, but they are called menopause mood swings.

Prior to perimenopause, your hormones work in harmony by co-existing with one another in a certain ratio. They are said to be balanced. This keeps your body healthy and functioning.

During perimenopause, the ratio of estrogen to progesterone significantly changes. Your ovaries produce less estrogen and progesterone than they did prior to perimenopause.

While estrogen levels fall from their pre-perimenopause levels during perimenopause, progesterone levels fall further. In terms of the ratio between them, there is greater percentage of estrogen in your body, relative to progesterone. There is an imbalance between them, when compared to their pre-perimenopause levels.

The imbalance between estrogen and progesterone makes you prone to mood swings. Estrogen has an excitatory effect (increases brain activity), (12) in your body. Progesterone has a sedative effect (calming). (13)

A higher level of estrogen relative to progesterone makes you more prone to mood swings during perimenopause. But....there is more.

A change in the levels of estrogen and progesterone affects the levels of the neurotransmitters.

There are two types of neurotransmitters .... Neurotransmitters that "excitatory" (revs up the brain cells) and neurotransmitters that are calming. The most well-known excitatory neurotransmitter is adrenaline. The most well-known calming neurotransmitter is serotonin. During perimenopause there is an increase in the levels of excitatory neurotransmitters and a decrease in the levels of neurotransmitters that are calming.

Changes in the levels of estrogen, progesterone and neurotransmitters are the cause of mood swings during menopause.

As mood swings during menopause are triggered by an imbalance between estrogen and progesterone, which causes the levels of neurotransmitters to change, the most effective way to relieve them is to re-balance the levels of estrogen and progesterone in your body. This involves taking bioidentical hormones.

However, many women are averse to hormone therapy of any kind.

Another effective treatment for mood swings during menopause is Cognitive Behavioral Therapy (CBT). (27) Controlled medical trials have found that CBT effectively relieves menopause mood swings...and improves quality of life.

It is a therapy that trains people to use techniques that help them control and manage their symptoms better, which is done in three effective ways (see page 55).

CBT trains people to use techniques that help them control and even prevent serious mood swings. CBT does not prevent the occurrence of mood swings. It reduces the severity of mood swings and the impact that they have on you.

Medical trials have found that CBT also relieves hot flashes, night sweats, anxiety, depression and insomnia.

12

You Are Not Going Crazy ... It's Menopause

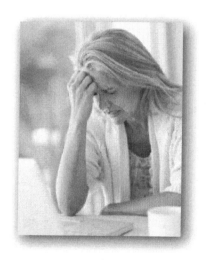

"I do feel as if I'm going off the deep end with this meno-pausal depression. My anxiety level is off the charts, I don't sleep well at night, don't function very well during the day. Just want to stay in bed with the covers over my head...Am I losing my mind?"

D. S.

More menopausal women experience hot flashes that any other single symptom.

However, if you were to group together the mental and emotional symptoms of menopause, into one category of symptom and call it "the menopause brain symptom", it would win hands down as the most prolific symptom. It would also be the most debilitating and life changing symptom.

Here is a small selection of quotes from women about their mental and emotional symptoms:

"I'm fine one minute .... Then out of nowhere I become this evil, vile mad woman..."

"Mood swings have completely changed my life. For me it ranges from the rage that I cannot control to total despair to happy again..."

"I am finding that menopause has catapulted me into depression! The flashes I can deal with, the night sweats etc. They're nasty, but I can deal with them. But the depression is unbearable..."

"Out of the blue three weeks ago I awoke with a complete feeling of fear and anxiety which has been getting progressively worse. As soon as I am awake I have a racing mind, feelings of doom, and a feeling of 'unease' which stays all day..."

The primary cause of all of the mental and emotional symptoms is a change in the chemistry of your brain during menopause. Menopause is a time of chemical upheaval in your body.

It would actually be more appropriate to say that these are symptoms of perimenopause .... As they disappear in post menopause.

They disappear shortly after a woman reaches menopause (no period for 12 consecutive months) for most women. Some women continue to experience some of these symptoms for several years during post menopause.

The trigger that causes a change in your brain chemistry during perimenopause is a change in the levels of estrogen and progesterone ... and a change in the ratio between them.

Prior to perimenopause, all of the chemicals in your body work in harmony by co-existing with one another in a certain ratio. The chemicals are hormones and neurotransmitters. They are said to be balanced. This keeps your body healthy and functioning.

The changing ratio between estrogen and progesterone disturbs the balance between all of the hormones and all of the neurotransmitters in your body. This is the primary cause of all of your mental and emotional symptoms.

A secondary cause of your mental and emotional symptoms is stress. Most women experience higher levels of stress during perimenopause, than prior to it.

Stress changes the ratio of the hormones and neurotransmitters in your body even further. The hormone associated with stress is cortisol. The level of cortisol in your body rises, when you experience stress. This exacerbates your symptoms.

There are two kinds of neurotransmitters – inhibitory and excitatory. (47) Excitatory stimulate your brain. Those that calm your brain and help create balance are called inhibitory. Inhibitory neurotransmitters balance mood and are easily depleted when the excitatory neurotransmitters are overactive.

High levels of certain neurotransmitters can enhance your cognitive responses (clarity of thought, memory, concentration, and learning), but worsen your emotional responses. Low levels of certain neurotransmitters can impair your cognitive responses, but improve your emotional responses.

When you experience stress, your body automatically goes into a hard-wired inbuilt survival mechanism called "fight or flight", (48) to help you deal with a threat. Your body produces increased amounts of certain neurotransmitters and decreased amounts of other neurotransmitters.

Norepinephrine is a neurotransmitter linked to the stress response. It is an excitatory neurotransmitter. Your brain increases the level of norepinephrine when you are confronted with stress. It makes you more alert. It helps you to think clearer and faster. It improves concentration.

But a high level of this neurotransmitter is also associated with increased sleep problems, anxiety and panic attacks.

Serotonin and GABA are also neurotransmitters associated with the stress response. They are calming neurotransmitters. In the stress response their levels are reduced...to enable norepinephrine to rev you up to deal with the threat.

As calming transmitters, serotonin and GABA play an important role in regulating memory and learning. Low levels of these neurotransmitters impede your memory and ability to learn. They are also associated with depression, anxiety, poor memory, inability to concentrate, and disturbed sleep.

When you feel stressed, your body has higher levels of norepinephrine than serotonin and GABA. When you calm down, your body has higher levels of serotonin and GABA than norepinephrine.

Balanced levels of neurotransmitters are needed for optimum cognitive and emotional responses.

If you have been experiencing increased levels of stress during menopause, the levels of these neurotransmitters will be out of whack.

To restore the neurotransmitter balance you must re-balance your hormones and reduce the stress level.

As the primary cause of neurotransmitter imbalance is hormonal imbalance, you must restore hormonal imbalance as your first step.

Restoring hormonal balance will not just relieve your mental and emotional symptoms. It will relieve all of your symptoms, because they are all caused by hormone imbalance.

Your hormones can be re-balanced by using bio-identical hormone therapy (BHRT) or by using bio-identical natural progesterone therapy.

Re-balancing your hormones, in itself, will reduce the level of stress you experience. But you should also regularly use a stress reduction technique to keep stress to a minimum. Embrace yoga, meditation, relaxation therapy or some other stress reduction technique regularly to keep stress at bay.

13

Menopause Depression: When Sadness Is So
Persistent That You Don't Want To Get Out Of Bed

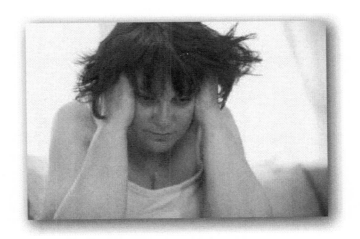

"Evelyn stared into the empty ice cream carton and wondered where the smiling girl in the school pictures had gone."

FANNIE FLAGG, FRIED GREEN TOMATOES
AT THE WHISTLE STOP CAFE

Dawn is my patient. She first started experiencing menopause symptoms two years ago. A few days ago I received an email from her in which she said:

"I just don't have the energy or enough desire or maybe even the ability to think and plan what to do. My house has gone to pot. I don't enjoy much. Takes everything in me just to make myself do the dishes or laundry, much less think about anything fun. I feel like I am watching the world from behind glass..."

She said that she wanted to alert me about what was going on with her, prior to her next appointment with me.

This is the first time that she has spoken about this kind of experience. What Jane has described is depression. (50) It is quite common during menopause. Menopausal women are up to four times more likely to experience it, than other women.

Many women experience menopause depression, but are unaware that they are depressed; others are in denial about it.

You may be suffering from menopause depression if you experience some of the following symptoms:

- Sadness and feeling weepy.
- Lethargy
- A loss of interest in things and activities you used to enjoy.
- Wanting to hide away from people, perhaps even by staying in bed.
- Constant tiredness and problems sleeping.
- Feeling that you cannot cope.
- Inability to see any glimmer of a 'light at the end of the tunnel'.
- You have to force yourself to do things. Each little action feels like climbing a dozen flights of stairs.

A key sign of depression (50) during menopause is either depressed mood or loss of interest in activities you once enjoyed.

Depression, if it happens, occurs most frequently during perimenopause. It abates in post menopause for most women.

Some women may have experienced depression prior to perimenopause. They are prone to experiencing depression during menopause. However the majority of women who experience menopause depression are experiencing depression for the first time.

Prior to perimenopause, your hormones work in harmony by co-existing with one another in a certain ratio. They are said to be balanced. This keeps your body healthy and functioning.

During perimenopause, the ratio of estrogen to progesterone significantly changes. Your ovaries produce less estrogen and progesterone than they did prior to perimenopause.

Changes in the levels of estrogen and progesterone disturb the levels of two neurotransmitters chemicals, adrenaline and serotonin in your brain.

Menopause depression is linked to insufficient levels of adrenaline and disturbed levels of serotonin.

Changes in the levels of estrogen, progesterone and neurotransmitters are the cause of menopause depression. (35)

Unfortunately, Doctors too often prescribe anti depression drugs on women who suffer depression during menopause.

Many doctors are not aware that depression is a common symptom of menopause. Antidepressant drugs cost Americans $11 billion each year and have many common side effects including sleep disturbances, nausea, tremors, and changes in body weight. Up to two-thirds of people with depression do not respond to anti-depressants. (51)

As menopause depression is triggered by an imbalance between estrogen and progesterone, which causes the levels of neurotransmitters to change, the most effective way to relieve it is to re-balance the levels of estrogen and progesterone in your body. This involves taking bioidentical hormones.

However, many women are averse to hormone therapy of any kind.

Another effective treatment for menopause depression is Cognitive Behavioral Therapy (CBT). Controlled medical trials have found that CBT effectively relieves depression...and improves quality of life. (22)

There are also online courses you can do. One such course is called "Beating the Blues". It consists of a 15-minute introductory video and eight 1-hour interactive computer sessions. (52)

Studies have found that all 3 methods are effective in relieving depression.

Researchers have found that CBT can reduce symptoms of depression in people who fail to respond to drug treatment. One study found that CBT is more effective in relieving depression than anti-depressants. Half the 234 subjects of the study who received CBT reported a reduction of symptoms. (53)

The North American Menopause Society (NAMS) reported that the studies found that CBT achieved a reduction in frequency and severity associated with hot flashes, depression, anxiety, and an overall improvement in quality of life.

They said that CBT was found to be effective for healthy premenopausal and postmenopausal women, as well as women with menopausal symptoms induced or exacerbated by breast cancer treatments. (23)

14

How Your Thyroid Impacts Your Emotional State
During Menopause

Is it menopause....or my thyroid....or what?
Did you know that it takes your mouth, esophagus, stomach, small intestine, large intestine, gallbladder, pancreas and liver just to digest a glass of milk?

The human digestive system is a series of organs that converts food into essential nutrients that are absorbed into the body and moves the unused waste material out of the body. It is essential to good health because if the digestive system shuts down, the body cannot be nourished or rid itself of waste.

Your digestive system is but one of ten major systems of your body. The major systems of the human body are:

- Skeletal system
- Muscular system
- Nervous system
- Respiratory system
- Cardiovascular system
- Digestive system
- Excretory system
- Endocrine system
- Immune system
- Reproductive system

All of the systems of your body depend upon the metabolism of your body. Metabolism is *all the chemical processes going on continuously inside your body that allow life and normal functioning.*

Your metabolism has two parts, which are carefully regulated by the body to make sure they remain in balance (54):

1. Catabolism – Catabolism is the breaking down of things. It is the part of metabolism that breaks down food components (such as carbohydrates, proteins and fats) into their simpler forms, which can then be used to create energy and provide the basic building blocks needed for growth and repair.
2. Anabolism – Anabolism is the building up of things. It is the part of metabolism in which our body is built or repaired. Anabolism requires energy that ultimately comes from our food. When we eat more than we need for daily anabolism, the excess nutrients are typically stored in our body as fat.

Your thyroid gland regulates your metabolism. (55) It produces your thyroid hormones. The two main thyroid hormones are triiodothyronine (known as T3) and thyroxine (known as T4).

Thyroxine plays a key role in determining how fast or slow the chemical reactions of metabolism proceed in your body. It is known as the metabolism hormone.

Menopause has a major impact on thyroxine levels, causing debilitating symptoms in 26% of menopausal women.

Perimenopause is a time of the greatest hormonal upheaval in your body. Prior to perimenopause, all of the hormones in your body work in harmony by co-existing with one another in a certain ratio. They are said to be balanced. This keeps your body healthy and functioning.

During perimenopause, the ratio of estrogen to progesterone significantly changes. There is more estrogen relative to progesterone.

While estrogen is generally falling, their levels fluctuate. The level of progesterone falls continuously. There is insufficient progesterone in your body to counter-balance the levels of estrogen in your body.

The changing ratio between estrogen and progesterone disturbs the balance between all of the other hormones in your body. This is the trigger that causes all of your menopause symptoms.

Thyroid levels can become high (hyperthyroidism) or low (hypothyroidism). Hyperthyroidism is commonly called over-active thyroid, while hypothyroidism is commonly called under-active thyroid.

Hypothyroidism is the predominant condition, affecting 26% of menopausal women. (56) It is a condition in which there is insufficient thyroid hormone levels to efficiently manage the metabolism.

SYMPTOMS OF HYPOTHYROIDISM

Many of the symptoms of menopause are also symptoms of hypothyroidism. Some common symptoms of hypothyroidism include:

- Exhaustion
- Brain fog
- Poor memory
- Depression
- Fatigue
- Mood swings
- Low energy level
- Dry skin
- Hair loss
- Sleep Disturbance
- Anxiety
- Nervousness
- Heart Palpitations

TREATING HYPOTHYROIDISM

Because the symptoms of hypothyroidism and menopause are similar, doctors often misdiagnose hypothyroidism symptoms as menopause symptoms. They prescribe conventional HRT, antidepressants, or sleeping pills — which miss the real problem entirely, or even make symptoms worse.

If you take conventional HRT for a hypothyroid condition, you will worsen the condition and your symptoms. The major component of conventional HRT is estrogen. As your body already has too much estrogen relative to progesterone, taking conventional HRT causes further hormone imbalance and destabilizes thyroid hormones even further.

To relieve symptoms of hypothyroidism, your hormones must be re-balanced.

You must increase the level of progesterone and decrease the levels of estrogen in your body. Increased levels of progesterone in your body will reduce your levels of estrogen. When estrogen and progesterone are re-balanced, it will trigger a natural process in your body that will bring your thyroid hormones, as well as all of your other hormones, back into balance.

As mentioned earlier, your hormones can be re-balanced by using bio-identical hormone therapy (BHRT) or by using bio-identical natural progesterone therapy.

If your doctor attempts to treat your hypothyroid condition just by increasing the levels of your thyroid hormones, it will not relieve your symptoms nor cure the condition. The underlying cause of the condition during menopause is too little progesterone in your body relative to estrogen. The cause must be addressed to cure the condition.

15

Why Stress Is Your Worst Enemy During Menopause

"There cannot be a stressful crisis next week. My schedule is already full."

HENRY KISSINGER

Menopause is the most stressful phase of a woman's life. It is a time when all of the hormone levels in your body are changing. Your changing hormone levels are triggering an upheaval in all of the systems of your body. This is the cause all of your menopause symptoms.

If you are encountering moderate to severe symptoms, your symptoms are causing you to experience mental, emotional and physical stress.

Stress exacerbates every menopause symptom.

If you suffer with moderate to severe symptoms, such as hot flashes, joint pain, depression, anxiety, disturbed sleep, weight gain, memory loss or any other symptom, stress **is** making your symptoms worse. The more stress you experience, the worse your symptoms will be.

The symptom that troubles a majority of menopausal woman is hot flashes. A study (57) was conducted to determine the effect that stress has on hot flashes. The researchers found the following:

- Women who rated themselves as "moderately anxious", due to life stresses, experienced three times as many hot flashes compared with women who were within "normal" anxiety range.
- Women with "high" anxiety scores experienced five times as many hot flashes.

WHAT IS STRESS?

Stress is difficult to define because it is subjective. What causes you to feel stress during menopause may not cause another woman to feel stress ... and vice versa. Having said that, here is a definition of stress that I favor:

"Stress is a feeling of anxiety and tension brought about by anything that you perceive to be a threat to your well-being. It is a physiological, mental and emotional reaction to that threat."

The most important word in the above definition is *"perceive"*. The definition of perceive is *"to interpret or regard someone or something in a particular way."*

If you experience severe and/or frequent menopause symptoms, you probably perceive them as a threat to your well-being. Per the definition of stress above, they will be a stressful experience for you ... for as long as you regard them in that way

Stress has a close cousin. It is anxiety. Anxiety is defined as a feeling of worry, nervousness, or unease about something with an uncertain outcome.

Stress and anxiety go hand in hand. Anxiety is most commonly triggered by the stress in our lives.

What is the difference between stress and anxiety? Stress is a reaction to something happening now. Anxiety is a reaction to something that is going to happen at a future date, may happen at a future date, or may never actually happen at all.

When you experience stress, your body automatically goes into a hard-wired inbuilt survival mechanism called "fight or flight", to help you deal with a threat, or perceived threat. It produces increased amounts of cortisol, which is known as the stress hormone.

Fight or flight is an automatic response mechanism that has evolved to help humans deal with threats, or perceived threats, to their survival. Here is how your body responds:

1. You are faced with stress.
2. A complex hormonal cascade ensues, and your adrenal glands produce cortisol.
3. Cortisol prepares your body for a fight-or-flight response. It
   - Floods your body with glucose (blood sugar) to give you a surge of immediate energy
   - Inhibits insulin production. Insulin causes glucose to be stored in the cells of your body, whereas it is needed for immediate use to deal with the stressful situation
   - Increases your heart rate
   - Decreases the performance of systems of your body that are not essential to deal with the stressful situation. i.e. – your metabolism (thyroid hormone) and your immune system
4. You address and resolve the situation.
5. Hormone levels return to normal.

If you experience moderate to severe menopause symptoms frequently, steps 1 – 3 of the "fight or flight" response can be engaged permanently, flooding your body with cortisol. Steps 4 and 5 may not occur. When this happens, stress has become chronic.

Chronic stress during menopause has the following effects on your body

1. Your glucose levels will be high continuously.
2. Your insulin level will be high continuously as your body attempts to remove glucose from your blood and move it into the cells of your body.
3. Your thyroid level will be chronically low …. possibly to the level of hypothyroidism (underactive thyroid).

These responses affect every system of your body. They will worsen all of your menopause symptoms.

If chronic stress during menopause is allowed to persist, it can lead to life threatening diseases.

Some ways to reduce stress during menopause:

- Any type of meditation will reduce stress and lower cortisol levels. Meditation is a practice of concentrated focus upon a sound, object, visualization, the breath etc. for an extended period of time. In so doing, your breathing slows down and your stress and cortisol level falls.
- Yoga will reduce stress. In yoga, the body, breath and mind are seen as key aspects of each and every human being. The system and various techniques of yoga, increases tranquility and clarity of the mind.
- Relaxation therapy reduces stress. It is a technique involving breathing therapy, which focuses on helping you relax each of your muscle groups and therefore achieving overall relaxation. You are shown how to do the technique so you can continue the therapy at home.
- Music has the power to improve mood and reduce stress during menopause. Listening to music that you love, and that fits whatever mood you're in, has been shown to lower cortisol levels.
- Having fun and laughing reduces cortisol levels. Research has revealed that cortisol is suppressed when you laugh. Try to find ways in your daily life to have fun, laugh and joke as much as possible and you'll lower cortisol levels and stress during menopause. (58)
- Increase your intake of vitamin B6, vitamin B5 (pantothenic acid), and vitamin C. These nutrients play an important role in your

body's regulation of cortisol levels. The levels of these nutrients are depleted by stress.

Additionally, if you eat right and exercise every day, it will help you to reduce stress during menopause.

16

How Stress Saps Your Energy And Makes You Feel Exhausted

"Worry and stress affects the circulation, the heart, the glands, the whole nervous system, and profoundly affects heart action."

CHARLES W. MAYO, M.D.

When you suddenly face danger or feel threatened in some way, you feel anything but tired. Your body automatically goes into a hard-wired inbuilt survival mechanism "fight or flight", to help you deal with the threat. It produces increased amounts of cortisol, which is known as the stress hormone.

The "fight or flight" response prepares your body for extreme action:

- Your heart beats more rapidly making you more alert.
- Your energy level increases to prime you to confront and deal with the threat.
- Body systems that are not essential to meet the threat ... i.e. digestive system, metabolism, immune system ... are downgraded in importance and performance until the threat abates.

The "fight or flight" response evolved as a short term response. Once the threat abates, cortisol levels reduce to pre- threat levels and the body systems that were "put on hold", so to speak, normalize.

For many women, the "fight or flight" mechanism is triggered more often during menopause, and less often at other time in their lives. What's more, it is "turned on" permanently for many women during menopause because of stress associated with menopause.

Stress is a feeling of anxiety and tension brought about by anything that you perceive to be a threat to your well-being. It is a physiological, mental and emotional reaction to that threat.

Menopause symptoms cause you to experience stress. They trigger the "fight or flight" mechanism. If your symptoms are moderate to severe and/ or frequent, the "fight or flight" mechanism may be activated permanently.

The definition of stress is an academic matter, when it comes to menopause. What is more important is to identify your stressors, those things that bring about your stress during menopause, and what you can do to reduce your stressors levels.

In a sense, you could think of your symptoms of menopause as stressors. However, what bring about stress are not so much your symptoms, but your reactions to those symptoms. For example:

- Mood swings can upset relationships. An upset relationship is the stressor.
- Hot flashes or night sweats disturb your sleep. Disturbed sleep is the stressor.
- Weight gain changes your physical appearance. Your physical appearance is the stressor.
- Memory loss embarrasses of frustrates you. Embarrassment or frustration is the stressor.

The "fight or flight" response to stress begins with increased production of cortisol by your body. Cortisol increases sugars (glucose) in your bloodstream to give you the energy you need to combat the threat.

It also curbs functions in your body that are non-essential or detrimental in a fight-or-flight situation….like your metabolic system, immune system and digestive system etc.

When you feel a great deal of stress, your cortisol level can remain high for an extended period of time. This curtails the functioning of your other body systems for an extended period of time as well.

Cortisol is one of three major hormones in your body that control most of the functions of your body. The other two are insulin and thyroid hormones. High levels of cortisol have a big impact on the levels of the other two major hormones.

High levels of cortisol inhibit your body's production of insulin. (59) Your body's primary source of energy is glucose (blood sugar). When you eat, food is converted into glucose. Glucose enters your bloodstream. At the same time, your body produces insulin to take the glucose to the cells of your body, where it is stored for future use.

High levels of cortisol prevent glucose from being stored, favoring its immediate use. In addition, cortisol also stimulates the production of glucose by the liver. As a result, glucose levels typically rise within the bloodstream in response to cortisol. (60)

Glucose keeps you alert and provides you with energy to "fight or flight". This high level of "alertness" disturbs your sleep. Moreover, high levels of glucose in your blood, a condition known as insulin resistance, leads to diabetes and other illnesses.

The most common feature of insulin resistance is fatigue. It wears people out; some are tired just in the morning or afternoon, others are exhausted all day.

Stress and high levels of cortisol lead to hypothyroidism (underactive thyroid). As discussed earlier, thyroid regulates your metabolism. Think of your metabolism as the "boiler room" of your body. When thyroid functioning diminishes, it brings about the condition known as hypothyroidism. It is estimated that 25% of menopausal women experience hypothyroidism.

Fatigue is usually the first symptom mentioned in connection with hypothyroidism.

Hypothyroidism has also been linked to insulin resistance. Thyroid hormone plays a role in glucose metabolism, and numerous studies reveal how insulin resistance affects thyroid health.

17

Are You Experiencing Weight Loss Resistance?

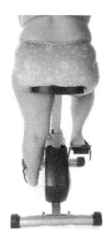

When daily exercise results in ZERO weight loss!

JUST A FEW OF WOMEN'S SAYS ABOUT MENOPAUSE AND
WEIGHT LOSS:

*"I am seriously in a panic state about my recent weight gain....Literally
NOTHING works anymore. I eat nothing but smoothies and salads and good
quality protein, no artificial sweeteners and I exercise every day ... but I've gained
20 lbs. in the last year."*

"I have weight gain round my middle now, despite eating a healthy diet-no sweets, chocolate or cookies. I eat plenty of salads, fish, veg, rice and some fruit. I just can't get rid of it."

"Menopause is causing my body to hang onto every last pound of fat... for what reason I do not know... I eat right and move a lot, gardening, walking, cleaning a big house, and I just can't lose a LB. Beyond frustrating."

"The old "calorie in, calorie out" theory does not seem to apply any more. Even with diet pills I have to just about kill myself working out daily to see any loss at all."

What these women are describing is a condition in which they have become resistant to weight loss.

Weight gain during menopause is the norm. 90% of menopausal women gain some weight between the ages of 35 and 55. On average, women gain 12-15 pounds during menopause. Many women gain much more than that. Around 30% of women aged 50 to 59 are not just overweight, but obese.

One of the most common concerns expressed by menopausal women is how easy it is to gain weight and how hard it is to lose weight (weight loss resistance).

A woman is weight loss resistant when despite her best efforts she cannot lose weight. Best efforts include:

- Following a recommended healthy diet for weight loss.
- Daily exercise.

No diet and no amount of exercise ... including working out at the gym ... bring about a loss of weight.

Weight loss resistance occurs when a woman has imbalances in one or more systems of her body. (62) Until imbalances are addressed, no amount of working out at the gym will fix it.

There are six systemic imbalances that contribute to weight loss resistance in women:

1. Imbalance in the reproductive system.
2. Imbalance in the digestive system.
3. Imbalance in the metabolic system.
4. Imbalance in the adrenal system.
5. Imbalance in the nervous system.
6. Imbalance in the immune system.

REPRODUCTIVE SYSTEM IMBALANCE AND WEIGHT LOSS

During menopause your ovaries produce less estrogen and progesterone, than prior to the onset of perimenopause. Not only do their levels change, but the ratios between them changes. Your ovaries produce more estrogen, relative to progesterone. Estrogen becomes dominant.

Estrogen dominance causes your body to store more fat than prior to perimenopause. It also makes it more difficult to burn fat when exercising

Your hormones are chemical messengers that control all the systems of your body. As your body functions as a holistic system, changes in one part of your body affects other parts of your body. Changes in the level of one hormone affect the levels of all of the hormones in your body.

DIGESTIVE SYSTEM IMBALANCE AND WEIGHT LOSS

The hormone that regulates your digestive system is insulin. Insulin breaks down the food that you eat and converts it into energy. It delivers the energy to the cells of your body and stores some of it as fat, as a future energy source.

Estrogen dominance disturbs the production of insulin by your body. Your body produces more insulin during menopause, than prior to it. As a result, your body stores more fat and make the burning of fat, during exercise, more difficult.

METABOLIC IMBALANCE AND WEIGHT LOSS

Your metabolism is regulated by the thyroid hormone. Estrogen dominance disturbs the production of thyroid by your body. The most common result is that your body produces insufficient thyroid ... a condition known as hypothyroidism. Hypothyroidism causes your metabolism to slow down. (56)

A slow metabolism = weight gain and difficulty losing weight.

ADRENAL IMBALANCE AND WEIGHT LOSS

Your adrenal glands produce cortisol, which is known as the stress hormone. Your adrenal glands increase the production of cortisol whenever you encounter stress (a threat to your well-being of some kind), to help you deal with the threat.

As menopause symptoms increase the levels of mental, emotional and physical stress that you experience, the level of cortisol in your body is higher during menopause, than prior to the onset of menopause symptoms. If you experience moderate to severe menopause symptoms, the level of cortisol in your body may be chronically high.

When your body produces too much cortisol, you get fat. Too much cortisol results in fat being stored around your waist. (61)

NERVOUS SYSTEM IMBALANCE AND WEIGHT LOSS

Estrogen dominance causes a change in your brain chemistry during menopause. It not only affects all of your hormones, it also affects the neurotransmitters, which as discussed previously, control all of your mental and emotional responses.

Disturbed levels of neurotransmitters cause you to experience negative emotions, which are associated with food cravings and bad eating habits. They also bring about emotions (depressed states) that are not conducive to doing exercise.

IMMUNE SYSTEM IMBALANCE AND WEIGHT LOSS

Many studies have examined the affect that falling estrogen levels have on the immune system during menopause. The findings of these studies are conclusive. Falling estrogen levels weakens the immune system during menopause. (63)

Inflammation is an immune system process by which your body's white blood cells protect you from infection with foreign organisms, such as bacteria and viruses. It's an essential, sometimes life-saving function of your immune system.

But over-activation of this healing response leads to chronic inflammation. Imbalance in the digestive system and the metabolic system are major causes of chronic inflammation. Chronic inflammation therefore is a significant source of weight loss resistance.

Weight loss resistance may be caused by a combination of any of the above 6 systemic imbalances, but one of them usually becomes prominent.

18

How Stress Prevents Weight Loss During Menopause

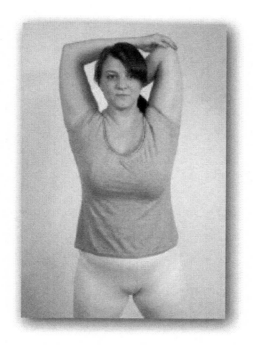

"I can't lose weight …. No matter how much exercise I do!"

H. T.

"Ambivalence is one of the biggest enemies of change. If you aren't sure that you really want to take action on something such as your weight, ambivalence will usually win."

LINDA SPANGLE, *100 DAYS OF WEIGHT LOSS: THE SECRET TO BEING SUCCESSFUL ON ANY DIET PLAN: A DAILY MOTIVATOR*

Are you unable to lose weight despite eating right and exercising every day?

You've got plenty of company. A large majority of menopausal women struggle to lose weight, after gaining weight during menopause.

There are several factors that prevent weight loss during menopause, despite eating right and exercising daily:

- Hormonal imbalance
- A slower metabolism
- Impairments in the digestive system
- Stress
- Impairment of the immune system

One, or more, of these factors is the principle factor that prevents weight loss during menopause. I have already covered how hormonal imbalance, a slower metabolism and impaired digestion prevents weight loss, in earlier chapters. However, the effect that stress has on weight loss during menopause is profound.

Before discussing how stress affects weight loss during menopause, it is important to understand why women experience higher levels of stress during menopause, than prior to it.

During menopause, stress levels are particularly high ... especially for women who experience moderate to severe menopause symptoms. Moderate to severe menopause symptoms are caused by acute hormonal imbalance, which causes an increase in mental, emotional and physical stress. High levels of stress are chronic for many women during menopause.

When you experienced stress prior to the onset of menopause symptoms, your body automatically went into a hardwired inbuilt survival mechanism called "fight or flight", to help you deal with a threat. It produced increased amounts of cortisol, which is known as the stress hormone.

In a nutshell, here is how your body responded: (58)

1. You were faced with stress.
2. A complex hormonal cascade ensued, and your adrenal glands secreted cortisol.
3. Cortisol prepared your body for a fight-or-flight response via the following:
    *   Flooded your body with glucose (blood sugar) to give you a surge of immediate energy.
    *   Inhibited insulin production. Insulin causes glucose to be stored in the cells of your body, whereas it is needed for immediate use to deal with the stressful situation.
    *   Increased your heart rate.
    *   Decreased the performance of systems of your body that were not essential to deal with the stressful situation. i.e. – your metabolism (thyroid hormone) and your immune system.
4. You addressed and resolved the situation.
5. Hormone levels returned to normal.

During menopause, if you are experiencing moderate to severe menopause symptoms, stress is continuously present. Your body reacts as if you are constantly under attack. The fight or flight response stays turned on. The long term activation of the stress response system results in an overexposure to cortisol.

Chronic stress during menopause has the following effects on your body:

*   Your glucose levels will be high continuously.
*   Your insulin level will be high continuously as your body attempts to remove glucose from your blood and move it into the cells of your body.

- Your thyroid level will be chronically low …. Possibly to the level of hypothyroidism (underactive thyroid).

HOW CHRONIC STRESS PREVENTS WEIGHT LOSS DURING MENOPAUSE?

When you experience chronic stress, your body produces too much cortisol continually. A high level of cortisol is preventing weight loss during menopause in 3 ways:

1. While you are eating right and exercising to lose weight, the high levels of cortisol will be adding fat around your waist. (61)
2. Chronically high levels of cortisol will keep your glucose levels constantly high. This will stimulate the production of ever-increasing levels of insulin in your body, causing your body to become insulin resistant, and reduce the capacity of your body's cell to utilize fat for energy, thus, increase your fat weight.
3. As discussed previously, high levels of cortisol decrease the level of thyroid hormone in your body. Thyroid hormone regulates your metabolism. Lower levels of thyroid means lower metabolic rate. With a lower metabolic rate, the capability of your body to burn fat reduces.

It should be clear now that if you do not reduce the level of stress that you have been experiencing, you will not achieve weight loss during menopause. While you do need to eat right and exercise daily to lose weight, you must also include a regular stress reduction technique in your life. This will help to modulate the cortisol level in your body, a key factor in achieving weight loss during menopause.

19

Insulin Resistance: The Most Likely Reason You Can't Lose Weight

"My weight keeps going up despite eating right and daily exercise. My body seems to want to hold onto every last pound of fat.... Despite me doing lots of daily exercise and eating right."

M. M.

I hear this so often. It seems to be the norm. There are reasons for it. When the correct reason is found and remedied, weight loss can occur.

The primary cause of gain weight during menopause is the changing levels of estrogen and progesterone in your body that begins with the onset of perimenopause and that carries on throughout your passage through menopause. It is also the primary cause of weight loss resistance.

Not only do the levels of estrogen and progesterone change, but the ratios between them also change. This creates imbalance between them.

Because your body functions as a holistic system changes in one part of your body affects other parts of your body, the changing ratios between estrogen and progesterone gives rise to changing levels of the other hormones. This in turn sets off changes to the levels of still other hormones ... and so on. This is what is called hormonal cascade. (64)

The end result is erratic production of all of the hormones needed by your body to regulate ... not only all your body systems, but specifically ... those systems that effect your weight management.

While the changing levels of estrogen and progesterone is the trigger that causes weight loss resistance during menopause, it is the changing levels of the hormone insulin, during menopause, that is the most common reason menopausal women find it hard to lose weight.

Insulin is a hormone produced and released by your body, when you eat. It breaks down the food you eat into glucose, which is commonly called blood sugar. Insulin directs the cells of your body to remove glucose from your blood and store it.

Glucose provides your body with energy, without which it could not function. Think of the relationship between glucose and your body, as being similar to gasoline and your car.

Think of insulin knocking on doors of the cells of your body. Those cells politely receive insulin's invitation and allow glucose in. With glucose in your cells, your cells can tackle important tasks such as growth, movement and repair.

Insulin levels rise in almost all women during menopause, due to the hormonal imbalance triggered by changes in estrogen and progesterone.

With more insulin in your body, your body tries harder to get glucose from your blood into the cells of your body.

However, once your cells have received enough glucose, they ignore the call from insulin to receive more glucose. Your body responds by producing more and more insulin, which is ignored by almost all the cells of your body.

There is one type of cell that listens to the call of insulin, your fat cells, which remain best friends with insulin. Your body can be either insulin sensitive or insulin resistant. (65)

If your body is insulin sensitive, insulin is doing the job it is intended to do ... the provision of glucose (energy) to the cells of your body.

If there is insulin resistance, your body will not be getting the "fuel" it needs. It is storing glucose as fat. Your body then produces increasing amounts of insulin, to try to give it the energy that it needs.

If you are insulin resistant, not only will you gain weight but you will be unable to lose weight....because your body will continually be adding fat.

All menopausal women are insulin resistant to some degree.

WHAT TO DO IF YOU ARE EXPERIENCING WEIGHT LOSS RESISTANCE DURING MENOPAUSE?

If despite your best effort, following a recommended healthy diet for weight loss and exercising daily, you still are experiencing weight loss resistance, and then try the following five step plan to enable you to lose weight:

1. Have the levels of your hormones tested to determine the extent of imbalance between them.
2. Re-balance your hormones.
3. Follow a proper diet that is based on physiological requirements for you.
4. Do not eat the 3 meals per day, as is customary. You should be eating something every 2-3 hours, during waking hours, to keep your blood sugar (glucose) in a normal range.

Eat a smaller breakfast, lunch and supper, than you have been accustomed to eating. In between each meal, and also after supper, eat a healthy snack...i.e. a piece of fruit, nuts, yogurt etc.

If you do not eat something every 2-3 hours, your blood sugar level will fall to a low level. It will then spike (rise sharply) when you next eat something (anything). This will greatly increase the level of insulin in your body.

5. Do at least 30 minutes of aerobic activity every day.
6. When possible add strength training to your exercise routine.

$$20$$

A Key That May Unlock Your Door To Menopause Weight Loss

"My body is holding on to fat...Why I can't lose weight? I eat well and I exercise daily"

T.L.

"We may not be able to control life's circumstances, but we always have a choice about how we use our minds to respond to them."

ELAINE MORAN

So you are overweight .... Maybe 10 pounds overweight, 20 pounds overweight or 30 pounds or more overweight.

You may be desperately trying to lose this weight. You may be following all the usual advice to lose this weight such as:

- Your diet is good.
- You are exercising regularly.
- You are doing a stress reduction technique regularly to keep stress at bay.

Still no weight loss, or worse, the pounds keep piling on.

An under-active thyroid (hypothyroidism) is a common cause of weight gain and inability to achieve weight loss during menopause.

Menopausal women are actually the group at highest risk of developing an under-active thyroid condition. 26% of menopausal women have an under-active thyroid condition.

Hypothyroidism is a condition in which there is insufficient thyroid hormone levels to efficiently manage the metabolism. Metabolism is the process the body uses to convert food into energy.

Most of us think of metabolism as the rate at which we burn calories. That's only part of the story. Your metabolism feeds the other systems of your body with the energy, oxygen and nutrients they need to function effectively.

A decrease in metabolism leads to a decrease in the flow of blood through your body. (66) Your blood carries energy, oxygen and nutrients to all of the cells and organs of your body. As your metabolism decreases, so does the supply of blood throughout your body. This diminishes the efficiency of all of the systems of your body.

It may be helpful to think of your metabolism as the "boiler room" of your body. As such, thyroid hormones affect nearly every cell, tissue, and organ in the body.

Therefore, when the levels of your thyroid hormones are low, your metabolism slows down. When your metabolism slows down, it affects your weight in two ways:

1. Your body does not use all of the calories ... from the food you eat ... for energy. It stores the calories not used for energy, as fat on your body (as a future source of energy), thus you gain weight.
2. Your body does not burn the fat on your body that it previously stored, when you exercise, thus you do not lose weight.

Furthermore, hypothyroidism causes insulin resistance. (67) As noted previously, Insulin resistance also prevents fat loss and weight loss during menopause. Regular exercise will not burn fat and you will not lose weight.

Also, hypothyroidism and insulin resistance increases physical and emotional stress levels. When you are under stress, your body produces cortisol ….known as the stress hormone. Protracted stress results in high levels of cortisol in your body. High levels of cortisol in your body cause your body to store more fat. It also prevents your body from burning fat. In the presence of high levels of cortisol, regular exercise will not burn fat and you will not lose weight.

HOW CAN YOU TELL IF YOU HAVE AN UNDERACTIVE THYROID?

The following checklist (68) has been compiled from details provided by the Merck Manual, the American Association of Clinical Endocrinologists, and the Thyroid Foundation of America. It will help you to determine if you have an under-active thyroid.

_____ *I am gaining weight inappropriately*
_____ *I'm unable to lose weight with diet/exercise*
_____ *I am constipated, sometimes severely*
_____ *I have hypothermia/low body temperature (I feel cold when others feel hot, I need extra sweaters, etc.)*
_____ *I feel fatigued, exhausted*
_____ *Feeling run down, sluggish, lethargic*
_____ *My hair is coarse and dry, breaking, brittle, falling out*
_____ *My skin is coarse, dry, scaly, and thick*
_____ *I have a hoarse or gravelly voice*
_____ *I have puffiness and swelling around the eyes and face*
_____ *I have pains, aches in joints, hands and feet*
_____ *I have developed carpal-tunnel syndrome, or it's getting worse*
_____ *I am having irregular menstrual cycles (longer, or heavier, or more frequent)*
_____ *I am having trouble conceiving a baby*
_____ *I feel depressed*

_____ I feel restless
_____ My moods change easily
_____ I have feelings of worthlessness
_____ I have difficulty concentrating
_____ I have more feelings of sadness
_____ I seem to be losing interest in normal daily activities
_____ I'm more forgetful lately

I also have the following additional symptoms, which have been reported more frequently in people with hypothyroidism:

_____ My hair is falling out
_____ I can't seem to remember things
_____ I have no sex drive
_____ I am getting more frequent infections that last longer
_____ I'm snoring more lately
_____ I have/may have sleep apnea
_____ I feel shortness of breath and tightness in the chest
_____ I feel the need to yawn to get oxygen
_____ My eyes feel gritty and dry
_____ My eyes feel sensitive to light
_____ My eyes get jumpy/tics in eyes, which makes me dizzy/vertigo and have headaches
_____ I have strange feelings in neck or throat
_____ I have tinnitus (ringing in ears)
_____ I get recurrent sinus infections
_____ I have vertigo
_____ I feel some lightheadedness
_____ I have severe menstrual cramps

If this checklist leads you to believe that you may have an under-active thyroid, ask your doctor for a TSH (Thyroid Stimulating Hormone) test.

The conventional normal values are between 0.35 – 5.0. When the TSH levels are within this normal range, it is assumed that the thyroid gland is healthy and functioning normally.

If the test confirms that you have an under-active thyroid, your doctor will prescribe thyroxine (thyroid hormone replacement therapy) to increase the levels of your thyroid hormones.

As the underlying cause of hypothyroidism in menopausal women is too little progesterone in your body relative to estrogen during menopause, the imbalance between estrogen and progesterone must be addressed as well … to achieve weight loss during menopause. If your doctor attempts to treat your hypothyroid condition just by increasing the levels of your thyroid hormones, it will not cure the condition. The imbalance between estrogen and progesterone will continuously disturb the levels of thyroid hormones in your body.

21

Menopause Flooding: Are You Afraid To Leave Your Home?

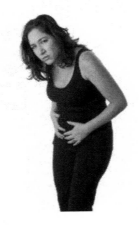

Am I going bleed to death?

Menopause flooding can be a scary experience the first time it happens. Women have said that they thought they were going to bleed to death, because of uncontrollable heavy menstrual bleeding.

"I had an unsettling thing happen. I stood up from a seated position and felt this gush of warm fluid. I ran to the bathroom and found that sure enough ….. I had had a sudden, large flood of dark red blood and large clots. I mean it looked like someone had been brutally murdered, there was that much blood." B. D.

I have just had the mother of all periods! The day it started I had arranged to have lunch with friends at a restaurant. Prior to going, I had a bit of warming, so I equipped myself by taking 2 pads with me…just in case. There I sat …. Chatting with my friends over lunch when the flood gates opened. I flooded right through my clothes and onto my seat. On my seat were large clots of blood. I have never been so embarrassed." J. C.

What these women experienced is called menopause flooding. It is the sudden onset of a very heavy menstrual flow… without warning.

It describes the sudden, unexpected onset of a heavy period … like turning on a tap. The blood can contain large blood clots that look like pieces of liver.

Normal menstrual protection is inadequate to deal with it. The easiest way to gauge whether you are experiencing flooding is to work out how often you are changing whatever form of protection you are using. For example, if you have to change your tampon or pad every hour or sooner, or if you frequently leak in the night, chances are you are experiencing menopause flooding.

Flooding is one of the menstrual symptoms women can experience during perimenopause. Collectively these menstrual symptoms are called irregular periods. Other symptoms include

- Infrequent period
- Too frequent periods
- Missed periods
- Painful cramping
- Abnormal duration of bleeding
- Changes in blood flow

Irregular periods can last anywhere from a few months to a few years. They end when you reach menopause (no period for 12 consecutive months). The severity of irregular periods depends on whether or not you treat the cause of this menopause symptom.

THE PHYSIOLOGICAL REASON FOR MENOPAUSE FLOODING

To understand the cause of menopause flooding requires some knowledge of the role of estrogen in the monthly menstrual cycle and ovarian aging.

Your body relies on a delicate balance of progesterone and estrogen. The balance between estrogen and progesterone is disturbed during perimenopause.

Although levels of estrogen fluctuate during perimenopause, their levels are generally 30% higher (69) than they were prior to perimenopause. Progesterone levels decrease during perimenopause.

Estrogen and progesterone regulate the production and shedding of the endometrium (uterine lining) during a menstrual cycle. (70) When the balance between them is disturbed, it can lead to the development of an excessively thick endometrium. This thickness contributes to more bleeding than usual.

In the normal pre-perimenopause menstrual cycle, estrogen encourages ovulation (the development of an egg) and causes the endometrium to thicken appropriately, in preparation for pregnancy.

As a woman gets older, the number of eggs in her ovaries decreases. When a woman reaches perimenopause, ovulation occurs less and less frequently. There are an insufficient number of eggs left in the ovaries to ensure that ovulation occurs every month.

During a perimenopause menstrual cycle, the body produces increasing amounts of estrogen in an attempt to bring about ovulation. This causes the endometrium to grow much thicker (71) than it does prior to perimenopause. If pregnancy does not occur, the body will shed the thick endometrium, producing the heavy menstrual period.

A SECONDARY CAUSE OF MENOPAUSE FLOODING

Many women say that menopause is the most stressful phase of their lives, especially women who are experiencing moderate to severe menopause symptoms.

Estrogen dominance triggers changes in the ratios and levels of all the other hormones in your body … including the major hormones insulin, cortisol and thyroid. It leads to erratic production of these hormones by your body.

Collectively … estrogen, progesterone, insulin, cortisol and thyroid hormones control and affect all of the systems of your body. The changes in the ratios and levels of these hormones disturb all the systems of your body, which is the cause of all of your menopause symptoms. When those symptoms are moderate to severe, they cause you to experience mental, emotional and physical stress.

Stress exacerbates flooding (72) because it lowers your progesterone level even further. When you are stressed, your body increases production of cortisol. When it increases cortisol production, it does so at the expense of progesterone production. The increased production of cortisol results in lower levels of progesterone.

DOES FLOODING OCCUR DURING ALL PHASES OF PERIMENOPAUSE?

No, it does not.

Dr. Patricia Kaufert, a scientist from Canada who has done one of the best studies about what women experience during perimenopause, found that women are likely to have a flooding menstruation just before their periods changed from regular to skipping. (73)

Dr Jerilynn C. Prior, MD and founder of The Centre for Menstrual Cycle and Ovulation Research (CeMCOR), has identified 5 phases of peri-menopause, and when menopause flooding is likely to occur. (74)

WHAT TO DO IF YOU ARE EXPERIENCING MENOPAUSE FLOODING?

It's always a good idea to have prolonged or heavy periods checked out by your physician, to eliminate the possibility of it being caused by disease.

If the cause is a disease, the disease must be treated. However it is rare that flooding during menopause is caused by disease.

If your menopause flooding is not caused by a disease, it is likely that your physician will recommend a surgical procedure to treat your heavy bleeding (75) such as:

- D&C (dilation and curettage) – D&C involves dilating the cervix and scraping the lining of the uterus.
- Hysteroscopy – This is a procedure in which a long, thin scope is inserted into the uterus through the vagina and cervix. It allows the doctor to see and remove fibroids or other growths that may cause bleeding.
- Endometrial resection or ablation – In this procedure, the lining of the uterus is removed or destroyed.
- Hysterectomy – This is the surgical removal of the uterus and cervix.

These invasive surgical procedures treat the symptoms of menopause flooding, not the cause. The cause of menopause flooding is too much estrogen in your body … and not enough progesterone.

There are two steps involved in treating the cause that you may choose:

1. Rebalancing the levels of estrogen and progesterone in your body. This is done with progesterone therapy, mainly through BHRT. Self-administered natural progesterone therapy increases the level of progesterone in your body, while lowering the level of estrogen.
2. Use one or more stress reduction techniques regularly (mentioned previously). This will lower your cortisol level and increase your progesterone level.

22

The Fire Raging Inside You During Menopause

"No one knows our bodies or our subjective experiences like we do. This means we can rest secure in our knowledge of ourselves and what we're going through, even when the medical profession doesn't understand or believe us...This means that no one can understand your life, symptoms, or illness like you can. This can be incredibly empowering: you are the expert. But, it also carries great responsibility: to live as happily and as fully as possible, you must listen to your body and trust your instincts."

SARAH HACKLEY

The journey through menopause ignites a fire that rages inside you. That fire is chronic inflammation. The literal definition of inflammation is to "set on fire."

Women are particularly prone to chronic inflammation especially during and after menopause. (76)

WHAT IS CHRONIC INFLAMMATION?

To understand chronic inflammation, you must first understand inflammation.

Inflammation is a body process that is vital to your health and well-being. It is your body's attempt at self-protection. It works to remove harmful stimuli, damaged cells, irritants, or pathogens (bacteria, viruses, or other microorganisms that can cause disease).

It all starts with the immune system, your body's first line of defense against any kind of harm. When you're injured or ill, your body dispatches white blood cells to root out the harmful stimuli and jump-start the healing process. When the threat has been dealt with, the inflammation process ends.

But the inflammation process also has a quiet, dark side, **chronic inflammation.** (77) Chronic "hidden" inflammation occurs throughout your body when something kick-starts the immune system and disengages the shut-off button. The white blood cells are mobilized and they end up just hanging around, often for a long, long time. The white blood cells attack healthy tissue and causing it to degrade.

While you not aware of it chronic inflammation is hidden in, but you will become aware of its consequences in due course. You won't feel pain or feel sick initially, but a fire is quietly smoldering within you, upsetting the delicate balance among all of the systems of your body.

THE LINK BETWEEN MENOPAUSE AND CHRONIC INFLAMMATION

Your body is a holistic system ... its parts are interconnected. All of the parts of your body are controlled by your hormones. Hormones are chemical messengers that direct your body to perform specific tasks.

Prior to perimenopause, all of the hormones in your body work in harmony by co-existing with one another in a certain ratio. They are said to be balanced. This keeps your body healthy and functioning.

However, estrogen dominance triggers changes in the ratios and levels of all the other hormones in your body, including the major hormones insulin, cortisol and thyroid. It leads to erratic production by your body of these hormones.

Collectively, estrogen, progesterone, insulin, cortisol and thyroid hormones control and affect all of the systems in your body. The changes in the ratios and levels of these hormones disturb all the systems of your body, resulting in chronic inflammation.

Menopause causes a domino effect in your body. A domino effect is the cumulative effect produced when one event sets off a chain of similar events.

Menopause begins in your ovaries. It ends having affected every part of your body. It affects the following:

- Circulatory system
- Nervous system
- Digestive system
- Respiratory system
- Immune system
- Urinary system
- Endocrine system
- Lymphatic system
- Skeletal system
- Muscular system
- Integumentary system
- Reproductive system

THE LINK BETWEEN CORTISOL, INSULIN, THYROID AND CHRONIC INFLAMMATION

During menopause many women experience stress levels that are particularly high … especially women who experience moderate to severe menopause symptoms. Moderate to severe menopause symptoms are caused by acute hormonal imbalance, which causes an increase in mental, emotional and physical stress. High levels of stress are chronic for many women during menopause.

When you experience stress, your body automatically goes into a hardwired inbuilt the "fight to fight "survival mechanism, to help you deal with a threat. It produces increased amounts of cortisol, which is known as the stress hormone.

Chronic stress (chronically high levels of cortisol) during menopause has the following effects on your body:

1. Your glucose levels will be high continuously.
2. Your insulin level will be high continuously as your body attempts to remove glucose from your blood and move it into the cells of your body.
3. Your thyroid level will be chronically low possibly to the level of hypothyroidism (underactive thyroid).

High glucose levels in itself causes inflammation in your body. It also causes your body to produce excessive amounts of insulin, causing insulin resistance, which is inflammatory.

High levels of insulin reduces the level of thyroid hormone in your body, causing hypothyroidism (underactive thyroid), which is inflammatory.

HEALTH RISKS ASSOCIATED WITH CHRONIC INFLAMMATION

You may feel healthy, but if chronic inflammation is raging inside of you, then you are in trouble. You won't feel pain or feel sick initially.

However here are some of the diseases that it eventually causes:

- Cancer
- Heart disease
- Stroke
- Alzheimer's Disease
- Diabetes
- Arthritis
- Osteoporosis
- All autoimmune diseases

A FOUR STEP PLAN TO REDUCE YOUR RISKS FROM CHRONIC INFLAMMATION

1. First and foremost, rebalance the levels of your hormones as mentioned earlier. As it is, the changing levels of the hormones and ratios in your body during menopause are one of the chronic inflammation causes.
2. Follow a diet that is based on natural, fresh, organic and non-process foods, i.e., unprocessed meat, fish, milk, eggs, legumes, fruits, grains and vegetables. The less chemicals and process sugars entering the body system, the lower are the risks for chronic inflammation.
3. Do at least 30 minutes of aerobic activity every day. CV exercise lowers your cortisol level, increase oxygen supply and nutrients to the body cells, increase circulation and take away from the cells and organs waste products, all lowering probability for chronic inflammation.
4. Include regular stress reduction routines in your life. This will also reduce your cortisol level.

23

How Menopause Wreaks Havoc On Your Urinary System

I don't understand what is going on down there

Your urinary system is 1 of 13 major systems in your body that work together that enable healthy functioning of your body. When any of these systems malfunctions, it can result in death or disease. At the very least, it will have a negative effect on your quality of life.

Your body takes nutrients from food that you eat and converts them to energy. This is done by your digestive system. After the body has taken the food components that it needs, waste products are left behind in the bowel and in the blood.

Your urinary system removes waste products from your blood and prepares it for elimination from your body, in the form of urine. It is your body's drainage system for removing waste products.

In order for normal urination to occur, all body parts in the urinary system need to work together in the correct order. The urinary system (78) consists of the kidneys, ureters, urinary bladder, and urethra. The parts of the system work together as follows:

- The kidneys filter the blood to remove wastes and produce urine
- Urine passes from each kidney to the bladder through thin tubes called ureters

- Ureters empty the urine into the bladder, which rests on top of the pelvic floor. The pelvic floor is a muscular structure similar to a sling running between the pubic bone in front to the base of the spine
- The bladder stores the urine. When the bladder becomes filled, the muscles in the wall of the bladder squeeze, and the urine leaves the body via another tube called the urethra

There are two common urinary system conditions that arise during menopause, when one or more parts of the urinary system malfunction:

1. Urinary tract infections (79) a urinary tract infection (UTI) is an infection in any part of your urinary system, your kidneys, ureters, bladder and urethra. This is common in post menopause.
2. Urinary incontinence (80) a urinary incontinence (UI) is also known as "loss of bladder control" or "urinary leakage". This is common in perimenopause and post menopause.

Pelvic organ prolapse (81) is another urinary system condition that occurs during menopause. It is also prevalent during childbirth. The organs of the pelvic area such as your bladder prolapse from its normal place in your lower belly and push against the walls of your vagina. This can happen when the muscles that hold your pelvic organs in place get weak.

Urinary tract infections, urinary incontinence and pelvic organ prolapse (when it occurs during menopause) are caused by low levels of estrogen.

Low levels of progesterone also play a role. The level of progesterone in a woman's body falls continuously during perimenopause and is extremely low in post menopause. In post menopause your body still makes a small amount of estrogen, but it makes zero progesterone. Progesterone helps make estrogen receptors more sensitive. An estrogen receptor is a molecule in a cell that makes the cell sensitive to receiving estrogen.

When progesterone is deficient, estrogen receptors become less sensitive to estrogen. Thus, many women with sufficient estrogen will nevertheless have signs of estrogen deficiency, such as urinary system problems. When progesterone is restored to normal physiological levels, estrogen receptors become more sensitive and signs of estrogen deficiency disappear.

24

Don't Laugh, Cough Or Sneeze ....
And You Won't Leak

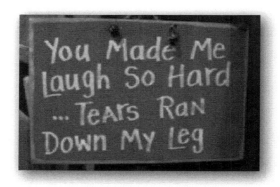

It is a universally acknowledged truth that statistics are dull, unless they are shocking.

Up to 57 percent of women between the ages 40 and 60 years old, and three-quarters of women 75 years old and older experience urinary incontinence. Experts suggest that many more women may have the condition, but remain undiagnosed because they haven't reported their symptoms to their doctor. (82)

According to the National Association for Continence, about 25 million adults in the United States experience urinary incontinence, and as many as half of them have symptoms that are severe and very bothersome. Yet only a third of those between the ages of 30 and 70 have discussed their bladder health with their doctors.

Urinary incontinence is a difficult condition to deal with emotionally. You lose control over what in the best circumstances can be an embarrassing bodily function. Feelings of humiliation, shame, and depression can cause people with incontinence to withdraw from friends and family, rarely venturing away from home or having anyone over to visit.

A recent survey of women suffering from incontinence (83) shows just how much impact it's having on lives:

- Almost two thirds of women feel embarrassed, anxious or nervous most of the time.
- 70% worry that they might smell.
- 60% say it affects their sleep.
- More than a third admits that it has caused relationship problems with their partner.

It is probably the most embarrassing of all the symptoms of menopause and women are ashamed to talk about it. They just pad up and die a little inside.

Urinary incontinence (UI) is also known as "loss of bladder control" or "urinary leakage". (80) You may experience it as a sudden urge to go, or leaking of urine, or frequent urination. You may experience all three.

UI occurs when the bladder and urethra are weakened to the point where they are unable to control urination, as they are intended to do.

There are two types of UI associated with menopause:

1. Stress incontinence – This is the most common kind of bladder control problem. Weakened muscles can't hold back urine when you cough, exercise, sneeze, laugh, or lift something heavy. The result can be a small leakage of urine or a complete loss of control
2. Urge incontinence – When your bladder muscles squeeze incorrectly or lose the ability to relax (so that you always feel the urge to urinate even when your bladder is empty), you may experience leaking or loss of control. This is sometimes called "overactive bladder".

Like all of the symptoms of menopause, UI is caused by falling estrogen and progesterone levels during perimenopause and low levels of both in post menopause. It is more prevalent in post menopause than perimenopause because their levels are lower in post menopause than perimenopause.

Healthy levels of estrogen strengthen the bladder and urethra. Low levels of estrogen causes a thinning of tissues of the bladder and urethra, which weakens them. They are unable to do what they were able to do previously.

A weakened bladder also leads to improper emptying of urine and higher residual amounts of urine left in the bladder.

A healthy level of progesterone helps estrogen to strengthen the bladder and urethra, by making their estrogen receptors more sensitive. An estrogen receptor is a molecule in a cell that makes the cell sensitive to receiving estrogen.

When progesterone is deficient, estrogen receptors become less sensitive to estrogen. Thus, many women with sufficient estrogen will nevertheless have signs of estrogen deficiency, such as UI.

When progesterone is restored to normal physiological levels, estrogen receptors become more sensitive and signs of estrogen deficiency disappear.

Urinary incontinence should not be considered normal or passively accepted.

You do not need to endure feelings of embarrassment and humiliation due to urinary incontinence. You do not need to restrict your activities because of it.

There are two things can do to reduce incidents of urinary incontinence during menopause:

1. Apply estrogen vaginal cream to your vaginal canal. It will strengthen the cells of your vagina as well as your bladder and urethra. (84)

It is safe because it is just applied locally to the vagina. Only about one percent of estrogen cream gets into the rest of your body's systems.

When using estrogen cream, it is advisable to supplement it by also using natural bioidentical progesterone cream. Progesterone will ensure that the estrogen is received and used by the cells of your bladder and urethra

2. Do Kegel exercises to strengthen the pelvic floor muscles that support and hold up the bladder. They are easy to do and it takes very little time. Essentially here is what you do....imagine that you are trying to stop yourself from urinating. Pull in and squeeze those muscles. Hold the squeeze for about 10 seconds, then rest for 10 seconds. Try to do three or four sets of 10 contractions every day.

25

How Vaginal Atrophy Affects Relationships In North America

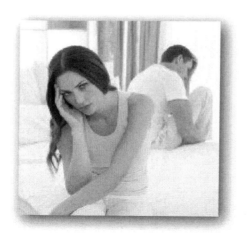

"When tough times come, it is particularly important to offset them with much gentle softness. Be a pillow."

VERA NAZARIAN, *THE PERPETUAL CALENDAR OF INSPIRATION*

An ongoing global survey of 4,100 postmenopausal women, who experience vaginal atrophy (VA), and 4,100 male partners of postmenopausal women, who experience VA, has been conducted in 9 countries.... to determine the effect that VA has on relationships. The survey is called CLOSER (Clarifying vaginal atrophy's impact On Sex and Relationships).

The objective of the study is to understand the emotional and physical impact of vaginal discomfort on postmenopausal women and their partners.

The findings of the North American segment of this study have just been released. The researchers examined the responses of 1,000 married or cohabiting North American postmenopausal women aged 55 to 65 years, with vaginal discomfort, and 1,000 male partners of those postmenopausal women.

Before I share the findings with you, it may be helpful if I provide you with some basic information about vaginal atrophy.

Vaginal atrophy is a condition in which the vaginal wall gets thinner and it gets inflamed. It occurs during menopause when there is a reduction in levels of estrogens. The symptoms of VA include vaginal burning, itching, dryness and irritation. Intercourse becomes painful because of it and it often leads to a decrease in sexual interest and activity. (85)

Women begin to experience vaginal discomfort during perimenopause. Declining levels of estrogen may cause the tissues of the vulva and the lining of the vagina to become thinner, drier, and less elastic. Vaginal secretions are reduced, resulting in decreased lubrication. (91)

As you approach menopause (final period), and during post menopause, you can expect the walls of your vagina to become thinner and more fragile — as well as becoming less elastic. The color becomes a pale pink, which reflects a lack of blood supply. It loses the quality of being open, expanded, or unblocked. This is caused by low levels of estrogen.

Findings of the CLOSER study (89)

- Vaginal discomfort caused 58% of the women to avoid intimacy.
- 64% of the women experienced loss of libido.
- 64% of the women experienced pain associated with sex.
- 78% of the men believed that vaginal discomfort caused their partners to avoid intimacy.
- 52% of the men said that their wife/partner experienced loss of libido.

- 59% of the men said that their wife/partner finds sex painful.
- Approximately 30% of the women and men cited vaginal discomfort as the reason they ceased having sex altogether.
- 56% of the women, who used local estrogen therapy to treat their vaginal discomfort, reported less painful sex.
- 41% of the women experienced more satisfying sex, as a result of using local estrogen therapy.
- 29% of the women said that their sex life improved, as a result of using local estrogen therapy.
- 57% of the men said that they looked forward to having sex because of their partner's use of local estrogen therapy.

Most conventional medicine and CAM (Complementary and Alternative Medicine) practitioners agree that estrogen therapy reverses vaginal atrophy and provides relief from it.

Conventional medicine practitioners will more often than not prescribe synthetic estrogen therapy to treat vaginal discomfort, in the form of a pill, cream, or vaginal ring. The pill taken orally enters the blood stream. It increases your risk of breast cancer. The cream or vaginal ring is inserted in your vagina. It carries a lower risk of breast cancer, because it is localized. It doesn't enter your blood stream. (92)

CAM practitioners are more likely to favor natural estrogen therapy.... bioidentical estriol therapy.... Taken as a vaginal cream to reverse vaginal atrophy and reduce its symptoms. Estriol is one of 3 estrogens that your body produces naturally.

Advocates of natural estriol therapy emphasize that it does not bear the health risks of synthetic estrogen therapy and that researchers have found that it actually protects against breast and uterine cancers. (93)

Natural or synthetic estrogen therapy taken as a vaginal cream will also act as a lubricant to reduce friction during intercourse.

It is also advisable to use a vaginal moisturizer. Moisturizers work, over time, to moisturize and strengthen vaginal tissues. They eliminate dry vaginal skin, protecting the vagina from irritation, itching, burning, and soreness, not only during sex, but throughout the day.

Regular sexual intercourse also helps to relieve vaginal discomfort. It increases blood flow to the vaginal area.

It is unfortunate that most postmenopausal women do not talk about their vaginal discomfort. Vaginal atrophy does not go away. In fact, it worsens if left untreated, according to Dr Wulf Utian, founding president of NAMS and a leading OB-GYN. (94)

$$26$$

The Little VD And The Big VD Of Menopause

"The basic conflict between men and women, sexually, is that men are like firemen. To men, sex is an emergency, and no matter what we're doing we can be ready in two minutes. Women, on the other hand, are like fire. They're very exciting, but the conditions have to be exactly right for it to occur."

JERRY SEINFELD

When you were younger, VD had one meaning …. Venereal disease. It was more of a concern to you when you were younger than it is now. For this reason I am calling it little VD.

The majority of menopausal women are in a permanent relationship. There is little risk of little VD when you are in a permanent relationship. One or both of you must stray for little VD to occur.

Many menopausal women who are not in a permanent relationship, experience a loss of libido during menopause. They are less interested in sex. Some have no interest in sex whatsoever. There is little risk of little VD for women in this category.

That leaves menopausal women who are not in a permanent relationship and who are sexually active. These women are at risk of little VD, if a condom is not used.

Big VD is vaginal dryness. Vaginal dryness is a common complaint of a condition called vaginal atrophy.

Vaginal atrophy is a condition in which the vaginal wall gets thinner and it gets inflamed. The symptoms of vaginal atrophy include vaginal burning, itching, dryness and irritation. The walls of the vagina become thinner and more fragile — as well as becoming less elastic. The color becomes a pale pink, which reflects a lack of blood supply. It loses the quality of being open, expanded, or unblocked. (85)

Approximately 40% of women experience vaginal problems during perimenopause and 60% of postmenopausal women experience them. Vaginal problems do not go away. If they are left untreated, they worsen. Dr Wulf Utian, founding president of the North American Menopause Society (NAMS) and a leading OB-GYN, says that by age 75, it's estimated that two out of every three women are affected. (86)

THE CAUSE OF VAGINAL PROBLEMS DURING PERIMENOPAUSE AND POST MENOPAUSE

When you were younger, the health of your vagina was attributed to a substance called Collagen. Collagen made up 75 percent of your skin, including the walls and tissues of your vagina. It gave structure to the walls and tissues of your vagina. It helped to keep them moist and firm. (87)

Since the age 30, you've been losing one percent of your collagen a year. The loss of collagen becomes more rapid in the first two years after menopause. 30% percent of your collagen is lost in the first five years after menopause. As a result, your skin loses its structure …. Its foundation … and what holds it together.

Science has long known that estrogen plays a vital role in maintaining the level of collagen in your body. The level of collagen in your body follows the same pattern as the level of estrogen, as you age. Falling estrogen levels = falling collagen levels. (88)

During perimenopause the level of estrogen in your body is falling from its level prior to perimenopause. During post menopause the level of estrogen in your body is much lower than it was prior to perimenopause.

HOW THE LOSS OF COLLAGEN AFFECTS YOUR UROGENITAL SYSTEM?

The urogenital system refers to those organs of the body involved with urination and reproduction.

A drop in collagen during menopause causes the vagina itself to become narrower and shorter. The walls of the vagina become thinner and less elastic. There is also a drop in vaginal lubrication. Women commonly report symptoms of dryness, itching, burning and general discomfort. In addition to day to day discomfort, a large study found that vaginal discomfort caused 58% of women to avoid intimacy. (89)

The loss of collagen weakens the organs of your urinary system (the kidneys, ureters, bladder, and urethra) and can bring about the following conditions

- Urinary incontinence is a common complaint. Weakened tissues of the bladder makes bladder control more difficult.
- Urinary tract infection (UTI) – A UTI is a condition where one or more parts of the urinary system become infected. UTIs are the most common of all bacterial infections. They result in eight to 10 million doctors' office visits each year in the United States.

A UTI is the most common bacterial infection in women in general and in menopausal women in particular. About half of all women will experience at least one urinary tract infection in their lifetime. For about 25 percent of these women, the infection will come back again within six months

- Pelvic organ prolapse is another urinary system condition that occurs during menopause.

As all of the urogenital atrophy conditions in menopausal women are caused by falling or permanently low levels of estrogen, the most effective way to reduce your risk of them is to increase the level of estrogen in your body. Apply estrogen vaginal cream to your vaginal canal. It will strengthen the cells of your vagina as well as the cells in the urinary tract. (90)

Estrogen therapy is the only known treatment for vaginal atrophy. It is safe because it is just applied locally to the vagina. Only about 1 percent of estrogen cream gets into the rest of your body's systems.

When using estrogen cream, it is advisable to supplement it by also using natural bioidentical progesterone cream. Your progesterone level falls continuously during perimenopause. In post menopause, your body still makes a little estrogen, but it makes no progesterone.

Progesterone will ensure that the estrogen is received and used by the cells of your urogenital organs. Progesterone helps make estrogen receptors more sensitive. An estrogen receptor is a molecule in a cell that makes the cell sensitive to receiving estrogen.

Whether or not you choose to use estrogen and progesterone, there is something else you can do to reduce your risk of urinary incontinence, urinary tract infection and pelvic organ prolapse.

There are several exercise techniques that will strengthen the organs of your pelvic area. These include Kegels, Pilates and yoga.

27

Do You Want To Be In "The Mood"?

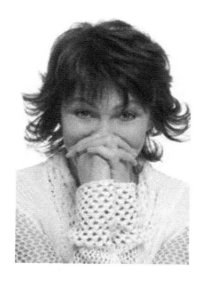

"If Sex is such a natural Phenomenon, how come there are so many books on the subject?"

BETTE MIDLER

LOSS OF LIBIDO

According to the North American Menopause Society (NAMS), (99) libido has 3 components:

1. Your sex drive, which is purely a physiological matter. It generally declines with age.
2. Your beliefs, values, and expectations about sexual activity.
3. Your motivation, which is your willingness to engage in sexual activity with a given partner.

As your sex drive likely has declined with age and as you probably have been experiencing some combination of menopause symptoms that has a negative effect on your mental and emotional states, it is hardly surprising if you experience a loss of libido, or a low libido.

Your libido is low if your lack of desire for sex causes stress or unhappiness for you. Dr Barb Dupree, MD, who was recently named the 2013 Certified Menopause Practitioner of the Year by the North American Menopause Society for "exceptional contributions" to menopause care, has said the following:

"If you're perfectly comfortable with your sex drive, you don't have low libido. But if you do have low libido, you're in the company of almost half of women over 40.

The ideal level of sexual desire is as individualized as a thumbprint. One woman's idea of low libido may be another woman's idea of nymphomania. The number of times in a week when you think about sex or pursue it is good to note, so you can notice increases and decreases in that number, but it's worthless for comparison with some national average.

If your desire is too low for your own happiness, then it is too low, and you may want to pursue ways of increasing it." (100)

Two new studies published in the journal Menopause offer hope to menopausal women who want to restore their libido.

An ongoing survey being conducted by the North American Menopause Society is showing that 79% of menopausal women have experienced a significant loss of sex drive during menopause.

Many women experience a decrease of libido during perimenopause. That decrease intensifies after menopause. One survey of 580 postmenopausal women, conducted by Siecus – the Sexuality Information and

Education Council of the United States, found that 45 percent of the women reported a decrease in sexual desire after menopause, 37 percent reported no change and 10 percent reported an increase. (95)

A study that examined the changes in sexual function, as women progress from early perimenopause to post menopause (96), found the following:

1. Women experienced a significant decrease in sexual desire during the late perimenopause.
2. Women using hormone therapy also reported higher sexual desire.
3. Those reporting higher perceived stress reported lower sexual desire.
4. Those most troubled by symptoms of hot flashes, fatigue, depressed mood, anxiety, difficulty getting to sleep, early morning awakening, and awakening during the night also reported significantly lower sexual desire.
5. Women with better perceived health reported higher sexual desire and those reporting more exercise and more alcohol intake also reported greater sexual desire.
6. Having a partner was associated with lower sexual desire.

For some women loss of libido is frustrating and they want to do something to improve it. For other women, it is a natural occurrence that leads to a pleasant transition in their relationship with their partners.

One study found that testosterone treatment increases libido.

Recent research on loss of libido found that testosterone plays a role in a woman's sex drive. Though present in only small amounts, some researchers believe that it has a significant impact on your sex life. While decreased levels of estrogen contribute to loss of sex drive during menopause, one of the leading researchers of testosterone treatment thinks that a decreased level of testosterone may be the main reason for it. (97)

Women at the age of 40 produce approximately half of the testosterone they did when they were in their 20s. Testosterone levels continue to decline with the onset of menopause or in women who have had their ovaries removed.

To date, the FDA has not approved a testosterone treatment for women. However, an important step toward developing a successful and safe treatment for women, after natural or surgical menopause, is to find out how much testosterone is really needed to bring desire back. Now a study has provided that and has confirmed that testosterone treatment increases libido.

The study found that women, who took a 25mg dose of testosterone weekly, experienced a significant increase in their libido. They had nearly three more sexual encounters per week after the treatment compared to before the study. (98)

It is important to note that taking 25 milligrams weekly boosted the subject's testosterone levels to five or six times what's considered a healthy level. This suggests that simply raising low testosterone levels to what's normal won't improve sexual function and these other measures.

The researchers said there were no serious negative side effects from taking this dosage. However, high doses of testosterone previously have been linked to negative heart effects. The researchers caution that cardiovascular and metabolic risks need to be investigated in long-term trials.

Margery Gass, MD and Executive Director of The North American Menopause Society said:

"Keeping hormone levels within the normal range for your gender and age is the safest approach. Hormones affect many systems in the body, and it takes a large and long-term study to identify side effects. One recent well-designed study in men reported that mortality was greater among older men taking testosterone. More is not necessarily better when it comes to hormones."

The other study found that flibanserin, a non-hormonal drug, increased libido.

This new study looked at 949 postmenopausal women with very low sexual drives. A little less than half of them were given 100 milligrams a day of flibanserin for six months. The others were given a placebo pill.

Those taking flibanserin reported increases in the number of satisfying sexual encounters and a higher score on a sexual desire scale, compared to those on placebo. About 38 percent of women on flibanserin said they experienced benefits to their sex lives after they took the treatment, compared to only 20 percent of the women on the placebo.

Thirty percent of the women on the treatment experienced side effects including dizziness, sleepiness, nausea, and headaches, but ultimately only 8 percent stopped the treatment because of them.

28

Scent of a Woman ..... During Menopause

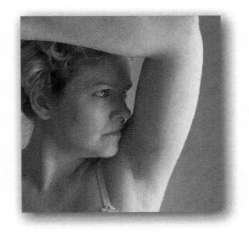

"Odors have a power of persuasion stronger than that of words, appearances, emotions, or will. The persuasive power of an odor cannot be fended off, it enters into us like breath into our lungs, it fills us up, imbues us totally. There is no remedy for it."

PATRICK SÜSKIND

Does your body odor embarrass you?
As if hot flashes and night sweats weren't bothersome enough, the sudden appearance of (or increase in) body odor can make you feel even more uncomfortable, more embarrassed and self-conscious.

Here is what some women have said about their body odor during menopause:

"I have noticed that my body odor is getting much, much stronger. I am really quite smelly under my arm pits. I shower daily have tried different deodorants etc. but nothing seems to be working. I have become so paranoid about people smelling me."

"I have suddenly developed an unusual, foul vaginal odor that is so strong that it penetrates my clothing and I can smell it myself. I worry that others around me can smell it as well."

"When I've been out running, I stink. I smell awful. A friend saw me running past her house the other day and came out for a chat – she must have thought I was mad because every time she came near I edged away a bit further."

"I often wondered why old ladies wore so much cologne…. I know and understand now!!! It's for the fear of smelling like a water buffalo!!!"

"I can sometimes hear the people at my work whispering and I know it is because of my body odor."

Menopause body odor (B.O.) does not usually get the same coverage as hot flashes or other expected menopause symptoms, but an increase in B.O. is common during perimenopause. Smelly B.O. is the proverbial elephant in the room. Though many women find it an uncomfortable subject to discuss, it cannot be ignored.

WHAT CAUSES AN INCREASE IN BODY ODOR DURING MENOPAUSE?

The increase in body odor during menopause occurs because you perspire more during menopause, than prior to it. Hot flashes, night sweats, and your other symptoms increase the amount that you perspire. They also increase the stress that you experience. Stress is a key ingredient of B.O.

B.O. is associated with sweat, which is the body's natural cooling system, but sweat does not smell. B.O. is a by-product of sweat. Bodies possess two types of sweat glands … eccrine glands and apocrine glands. They produce two types of sweat both of which are odorless. (101)

Eccrine glands, which are the main sweat glands, are located all over your body. They produce a more watery type of sweat, when compared to apocrine sweat. The primary function of eccrine sweat is to regulate body temperature.

Apocrine glands are located in the pubic region, armpits, mouth, feet and hair. They produce a thicker type of sweat, when you are stressed. It is a fatty sweat.

B.O. occurs when bacteria comes into contact with apocrine sweat.

Bacteria thrive in damp areas, the areas where apocrine glands are located. They feed on the fatty components of apocrine sweat and it is these bacterial by-products that cause a change in body odor during menopause. It is the cause of the following:

- Increased odor from your vagina
- Increased odor from your armpits
- Increased odor from your mouth (bad breath)
- Increased odor from your feet
- Increased odor from your hair

There are three kinds of sweat – sweat from heat, sweat from exercise and sweat from stress. Of the three, stress sweat is the hardest to control and gives off the foulest stench. Body odor during menopause is caused by stress sweat. Stress triggers the release of the thicker fatty apocrine sweat. (102)

Under normal circumstances, perspiration is meant to cool you down so you don't overheat. When it's hot or you're exerting yourself physically, your temperature *gradually* rises. Your body's internal thermostat, located in the hypothalamus, eventually recognizes that it better do something to chill you out and triggers the release of neurotransmitters that instruct millions of eccrine glands all over your body to produce sweat. As the sweat evaporates, it carries heat away from you, cooling you off.

It's a whole different story when you experience stress. Stress causes adrenaline and cortisol to rush into your bloodstream, raising your heartbeat and unleashing an ***instantaneous*** torrent of sweat from your eccrine glands and apocrine glands. The smell of stress sweat comes on real strong, real fast. (103)

Menopause body odor particularly intensifies as a result of hot flashes, night sweats, anxiety, panic attacks and mood swings. These symptoms are associated with increased sweating and stress.

Hot flashes and night sweats bring about an increase in perspiration that causes an increase in stress. Anxiety, panic attacks and mood swings bring about an increase in stress, which causes an increase in perspiration.

Other symptoms cause stress, but do not especially increase perspiration.

29

What To Do About Embarrassing Body Odor During Menopause

"I get out of the car, and I'm blasted by the stench of body odor. Cricket is beside me, and he's talking, but his words don't reach my ears.
Because it's my mother...Smelling...On my porch."

STEPHANIE PERKINS

It may be one of your worst nightmares!

Who wants to be told "you have awful body odor"? You're not alone. In one study, 46% of women said they'd willingly shave ten years off their life rather than be perceived as smelly. Another 76% said they'd rather gain weight than have chronic body odor.

Many women complain about embarrassing body odor during menopause. It makes them self-conscious. They wonder if others can smell the awful odor emanating from their body.

Some women become aware of their strong body odor (B.O.) for the first time in their lives during menopause. Other women are aware of their much stronger body odor during menopause, compared to their body odor prior to the onset of menopause.

Strong body odor is a symptom of menopause. It intensifies during perimenopause.

Your body produces a smelly odor when you experience stress and perspiration at the same time. Sweat alone does not smell. Stress alone does not create a smell.

As mentioned earlier, menopause body odor particularly intensifies as a result of hot flashes, night sweats, anxiety, panic attacks and mood swings. These symptoms are associated with increased sweating and stress.

Hot flashes and night sweats bring about an increase in perspiration, which causes an increase in stress. Anxiety, panic attacks and mood swings bring about an increase in stress that causes an increase in perspiration.

Other symptoms cause stress, but do not especially increase perspiration. Therefore they do not increase B.O.

Menopause B.O is caused by stress and perspiration that is associated with hot flashes, night sweats, anxiety, panic and mood swings.

As these symptoms are caused by hormonal imbalance, the frequency and severity of the symptoms can be reduced or eliminated by re-balancing your hormones.

Re-balancing your hormones involves taking hormones, otherwise known as hormone therapy. It is the only known way to eliminate menopause body odor.

However, many women are averse to using hormone therapy of any kind.

The most effective way to reduce body odor during menopause is to reduce the level of stress you are experiencing.

Stress exacerbates the menopause symptoms associated with B.O. Meditation, yoga, CV exercise, music are few of many stress reduction techniques which you could use.

There are number of other steps you can take to manage and reduce your body odor during menopause:

- Take a chlorophyllin supplement – Chlorophyllin is the water soluble derivative of chlorophyll. It has the unique ability of being able to bind to various odor causing compounds in the body. It neutralizes these compounds and removes them from the body.

- Wear cool comfortable clothes that breathe and dress in layers so you can control your body temperature better throughout the day.
- Change clothes more frequently, particularly after experiencing a hot flash.
- Bathe or shower more frequently paying particular attention to washing your armpits and genital region.
- Steer clear of dietary triggers like hot or spicy foods that can induce hot flashes or increase their severity.
- Eat a healthy diet.
- Use a stronger antiperspirant and deodorant.

30

Have You Got The Most Common Disease In America?

It's there all the time ... and getting worse

50% of adults in America have periodontal disease (gum disease), according to the Centers for Disease Control and Prevention (CDC). CDC is the leading national public health institute of the United States. (104)

Periodontal disease increases with age, 70.1% of adults 65 years and older have it.

Women are more prone to periodontal disease than men because of the hormonal fluctuations that they experience during various stages of their lives.

Periodontal disease is the most common cause of tooth loss among adults.

Menopause significantly increases your risk of periodontal disease.

WHAT IS PERIODONTAL DISEASE?

"Perio" means around, and "dontal" refers to teeth.

Periodontal disease is a chronic inflammation and infection of the gums and surrounding tissue. It is the major cause of about 70 percent of adult tooth loss, affecting three out of four persons at some point in their life.

The primary cause of periodontal disease is bacterial plaque – a sticky, colorless film that constantly forms on the teeth.

Toxins produced and released by bacteria in plaque irritate the gums. These toxins cause the breakdown of the fibers that hold the gums tightly to the teeth, creating periodontal pockets that fill with even more toxins and bacteria.

As the disease progresses, pockets extend deeper, and the bacteria moves down until the bone that holds the tooth in place is destroyed. The tooth eventually will fall out or require extraction.

In the USA twenty-five percent (25%) of all adults aged 60 years and older have lost all of their teeth. (105) A study conducted by the National Institute of Dental Research found that persons from 55 to 64 years of age had lost 1/3 of their teeth – an average of 10 teeth. A full set of adult teeth contains 32 teeth.

THE LINK BETWEEN PERIODONTAL DISEASE AND MENOPAUSE

Women are susceptible to gum disease, at times of hormonal imbalance, throughout their lives. Every significant change in hormone levels has an effect on the gums and on the other nearby tissues that support the teeth. However, the hormonal changes of menopause affect the gum health of women more permanently than the hormonal changes of puberty, menstruation or pregnancy.

While many factors can contribute to gum problems throughout the lifecycle, the most common cause of gum problems during menopause is decreasing estrogen levels. Research shows that estrogen levels can affect many oral tissues including the gums, salivary glands, joints, and jawbones. (106)

Decreasing levels of estrogen lead to changes in gum sensitivity, inflammation, and can mean a higher risk of periodontal disease.

Hormonal changes during menopause can result in different periodontal symptoms for each individual woman. Some women might experience heightened gum sensitivity, which can manifest as tenderness, pain, or irritation. Gum sensitivity can increase chances of developing a receding gum line, and women can experience gum infections or bleeding gums as a result.

Since estrogen also plays a role in regulating the immune system, when less of the hormone is present, the immune system may not be able to fight oral bacteria as well as before.

Estrogen deficiency after menopause is also associated with bone loss. Bone loss is associated both with periodontal disease and osteoporosis. A study found that bone loss in the alveolar bone (which holds teeth in place) was a major predictor of tooth loss in postmenopausal women. (107) Periodontal disease is the main cause of alveolar bone loss.

WHY YOU SHOULD BE CONCERN ABOUT GUM DISEASE?

The most obvious effect of gum disease is aesthetic – missing teeth. The way you look affects the way you feel. A recent study of over 3,100 adults aged 60 found that tooth loss appears to be linked to physical and mental decline in older adults. (108)

However there is a much greater concern. Gum disease is associated with and increases your risk of the following diseases:

- Heart disease
- Stroke
- Diabetes
- Cancer
- Lung disease
- Osteoporosis
- Autoimmune diseases

DO YOU HAVE GUM DISEASE?

Following is a questionnaire to see whether you suffer from gum disease:

1. Do you suffer from pains in the mouth?
2. Are your gums puffy and sensitive?
3. Do your gums bleed when you brush your teeth?
4. Do your gums bleed when you eat solid food?
5. Have gaps appeared between your teeth over the years?

6. Have your gums receded?
7. Do you have bad breath?
8. Have there been any changes in the overbite or the jaw correlation?
9. Is pus being secreted from the gaps between your teeth and your gums?

If the answer to any of these questions is yes, it is an indication that you have gum disease.

31

What You Should Do About Gum Disease During Menopause

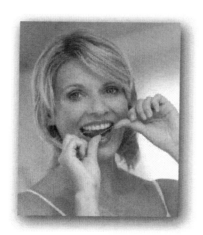

You can't cure it, but you can control it!

WHAT IS GUM DISEASE?

It is a chronic inflammation and infection of the gums and surrounding tissue. It breaks down the fibers that hold the gums tightly to the teeth and it destroys the bone that holds the teeth in place.

Six pertinent facts about gum disease:

1. Women are more prone to it than men, because of the fluctuating levels of estrogen that they experience during various stages of their lives.

Menopause significantly increases your risk of it, because falling levels of estrogen during menopause affect your gum health more permanently than the changes in estrogen levels during puberty, menstruation or pregnancy.

2. After menopause, your risk of it increases further. 70.1% of adults 65 years and older have it.
3. It is the most common cause of tooth loss among adults.
4. In the USA twenty-five percent (25%) of all adults aged 60 years and older have lost all of their teeth. (105)
5. A study conducted by the National Institute of Dental Research found that persons from 55 to 64 years of age had lost 1/3 of their teeth – an average of 10 teeth. A full set of adult teeth contains 32 teeth.
6. It is linked to many health problems in other parts of the body. A recent study found that people with serious gum disease were 40% more likely to have a life threatening chronic health condition as well. (109)

WHAT TO DO IF YOU HAVE PERIODONTAL DISEASE?

There is no cure for periodontal disease, but it can be controlled. If you control it you will reduce your risk of the diseases associated it. Here is what you can do to control it:

- Reduce plaque in your mouth – Plaque is the cause of gum disease.

Follow guidelines for oral health strictly. Brush your teeth and gums twice a day using an electronic, as well as a regular toothbrush. Use dental floss or an interdental tooth brush to remove food from between your teeth. Use a mouth rinse to reduce the amount of bacteria in your mouth

- Eliminate processed food from your diet – These foods contain added sugar, which becomes glucose in your blood after it is

consumed. A high level of glucose in your blood is conducive to plaque formation and a weakening of your gums.
- Do yoga, meditation, relaxation therapy or some other stress reduction technique regularly – Stress worsens gum disease.

When you experience stress, your body automatically goes into a hardwired inbuilt survival mechanism called "fight or flight", to help you deal with a threat. It produces increased amounts of cortisol, which is known as the stress hormone.

Cortisol increases glucose in the bloodstream to give you the energy you need to combat the threat. It also curbs functions in your body that are non-essential or detrimental in a fight-or-flight situation … like your immune system.

The higher level of stress during menopause contributes to a deterioration of your teeth and gums (110) in two ways:

- The high level of glucose in your blood is conducive to plaque formation and a weakening of your gums.
- A weakened immune system inhibits the fight against plaque forming bacteria in your mouth.

Ask your doctor to do a vitamin D test. Studies show that more than 1 out 2 menopausal women are vitamin D deficient. If the test shows that you are deficient, increase the level of vitamin D in your body.

Vitamin D deficiency is associated with gum disease because vitamin D increases calcium absorption and stimulates bone growth (periodontal disease erodes the bone that holds your teeth) and it is anti-inflammatory (fights infection).

A study of 11,000 subjects 50 years old or older showed that tooth loss was associated with lower levels of vitamin D. (111)

Consider estrogen therapy – falling levels of estrogen during perimenopause and low levels of estrogen in post menopause exacerbate gum disease. It weakens the bone in your mouth that holds your teeth.

If you are not averse to hormone therapy, taking bio-identical estrogen will help to stop the deterioration of the bone in your mouth. Unlike conventional HRT, taking bio-identical estrogen has no health risks associated with taking it.

32

They Told Me To Expect Hot Flashes ...
But Not Burning Mouth

"My mouth feels like it is on fire"

O. G.

It feels like my mouth is on fire. Every day when I wake it is fine. It gets progressively worse during the day. By the evening, my mouth can feel like it is scalding

This is what Olivia said, when I asked her how she was doing.

This is a common symptom during menopause that you don't hear much about. However, approximately 40% of women experience symptoms of Burning Mouth Syndrome during menopause.

WHAT IS BURNING MOUTH SYNDROME?

Burning Mouth Syndrome (BMS) is a hot feeling or sensation which can affect your tongue, lips, palate or areas all over your mouth. Sometimes it is called burning tongue syndrome. It is not a disease, but it describes symptoms.

Common symptoms of BMS include:

- Sore mouth
- Pain worsens as the day progresses

- A tingling or numb sensation in the mouth or at the tip of the tongue
- Dry mouth
- Itchy mouth
- Sticky mouth
- A metallic taste in the mouth
- Loss of taste/taste alterations
- Increased thirst

BMS usually begins spontaneously, with no known triggering factor. But some studies suggest that certain factors may increase your risk of developing burning mouth syndrome. These risk factors may include traumatic life events, stress, anxiety, and depression. (112)

The exact cause of BMS is not known. There are several possible causes of it, but because it is most common in menopausal women, researchers believe the primary cause is hormonal imbalance. (113)

BMS can affect anyone, but it occurs most commonly in middle-aged or older women. Women are seven times more likely to be diagnosed with BMS than men. The majority of BMS sufferers are menopausal women.

Also, as studies have found that traumatic life events, stress, anxiety, and depression are risk factors for BMS, these symptoms are abundantly present during menopause.

As discussed before, during perimenopause, the ratio of estrogen to progesterone significantly changes. The result is that during perimenopause there is more estrogen in your body, relative to progesterone, than there was prior to it. This brings about a condition known as estrogen dominance. (1)

Estrogen dominance triggers changes in the ratios and levels of all the other hormones in your body. As your hormones collectively regulate and control all of the functions in your body, the functions are disturbed. This is the cause of all of your other menopause symptoms….and it likely is the cause of burning mouth symptoms.

If your BMS symptoms are severe and affecting your quality of life, I recommend that you get your hormone tested and then with the guidance of a hormone expert, re-balance your hormones via the following:

1. Traditional HRT
2. Bio-identical hormone therapy (BHRT)
3. Bio-identical natural progesterone therapy

As hormone imbalance is the cause of all other menopause symptoms, and is the likely cause of BMS symptoms, you have nothing to lose and everything to gain by treating BMS as suggested above.

33

Are You Alarmed By Your Hair Loss During Menopause?

"Am I going bald?"

S. E.

Stephanie looked disturbed when she took a seat in my office. I was expecting her to talk again about her hot flashes, which had become more frequent and more severe. Instead she blurted out:

"Yesterday I almost died when I saw how much hair fell out in the shower. It swirled around my feet... It was a wad of hair the size of a mouse! I asked my husband if he'd still love me if I was bald."

Does it worry you when:

- Hair falls out in large clumps when washing it?
- Large clumps of hair appear in your brush or comb?
- You notice a visible thinning of your hair on the front, sides or top of your head?

If you are experiencing any of the above, you are in the majority, not in the minority.

Female hair loss usually begins at around the age of 30 and even as early as in the 20s or earlier. It usually goes unnoticed at this time. (114)

40% percent of women have visible hair loss by the time they are age 40, according to the American Academy of Dermatology. It gets even more noticeable during and after menopause.

By the age of 50, 50% of women will experience some degree of hair loss. Among post menopause women, as many as 65% of the women suffer hair thinning or bald spots. (115)

WHY WOMEN EXPERIENCE INCREASING HAIR LOSS DURING MENOPAUSE AND AFTER IT?

Hair loss during menopause, like all other menopause symptoms, is caused by changes in the levels of major hormones in your body. The hormones most associated with hair loss are the sex hormones estrogen, progesterone, and testosterone (testosterone is not just a male hormone ... a woman's body makes it as well, but in smaller amounts). Thyroid hormone and cortisol also play roles in hair loss.

As mentioned earlier, during perimenopause, not only do the levels of your hormones change, but the ratio between them changes as well. Generally, the levels of your sex hormones are falling, but some fall more than others. The level of progesterone falls continuously, while the levels of estrogen and testosterone fluctuate.

During post menopause, the level of estrogen in your body is low and the level of progesterone is zero. Your body still makes a little estrogen, but it makes no progesterone. Your ovaries continue to make testosterone after it stops making estrogen. (116)

To understand the effects that these hormones have on your hair requires an understanding of the cycle of hair growth and loss.

CYCLE OF HAIR GROWTH AND LOSS

Hair growth and loss occurs in a cycle that has 2 main phases

1. Anagen – this is the hair growth phase. Normally, hair grows about a half inch a month for 2-6 years, and then it goes into a resting phase.

Prior to perimenopause, approximately 85% of the hair on your head was in this phase

2. Telogen – this is known as the resting phase. You can think of Telogen as the shedding stage. Hair loss occurs during this stage.

Prior to perimenopause, approximately 15% of the hair on your head was in this phase.

According to MedlinePlus, which is a service of the U.S. National Library of Medicine and National Institutes of Health, the average scalp has 100,000 hairs and each person loses approximately 100 hairs daily. After a cycle of rest, the hair falls out and a new strand begins to grow in its place. (117)

True hair loss occurs when lost hairs are not regrown or when the daily hair shed exceeds 125 hairs.

HOW TESTOSTERONE EFFECT HAIR LOSS?
Testosterone is the hormone most associated with hair loss.

During perimenopause, testosterone levels fluctuate. The ratio between it and estrogen and progesterone can increase. (116)

Also, as stated previously, during post menopause your ovaries stop producing estrogen and progesterone, but they continue to produce some testosterone. When it does, it creates a condition known as testosterone dominance. There is too much testosterone relative to estrogen and progesterone.

A form of testosterone, known as DHT, is damaging to your hair and contributes significantly to hair loss during menopause. DHT causes your body to stop growing new hair. It curtails Anagen. This coupled with the shedding of hair during telogen results in an overall hair loss. (118)

HOW FALLING ESTROGEN LEVELS DURING MENOPAUSE AFFECTS YOUR HAIR?
Doctors know that hair thickens in pregnant pre-menopausal women due to increased levels of estrogen. Increased estrogen increases the ratio of

actively growing hair (Anagen) to resting hair (Telogen). The exact opposite happens to women after entering menopause. (119)

Prior to perimenopause, estrogen helps hair grow faster and stay on your head longer by maintaining longer periods of time in Anagen, the hair growth phase. Falling levels of estrogen during menopause, and low levels after menopause, results is a shorter hair growth phase (Anagen) and a longer hair loss cycle (Telogen). This contributes to hair loss.

HOW FALLING PROGESTERONE LEVELS DURING MENOPAUSE AFFECTS YOUR HAIR?

Progesterone functions as a natural DHT blocker. Prior to perimenopause, it protects your hair from DHT. During perimenopause and after that, low levels of progesterone makes your hair more susceptible to damage from DHT.

Progesterone has the following positive effects that help to stimulate hair growth

- Progesterone decreases the level of testosterone.
- Progesterone enhances blood flow enabling nutrients, needed for hair growth, to reach your hair follicles.

Progesterone is the main ingredient in many hair loss products. (120)

HOW TO REVERSE HAIR LOSS DURING MENOPAUSE AND AFTERWARDS?

First let me put your mind at ease. Natural baldness is a man thing. Women don't go bald naturally. Women who undergo chemotherapy may go bald.

As hair loss during menopause is caused by hormone imbalance, you need to re-balance your hormones to reverse your hair loss.

The most effective treatment for hair loss entails consultation with a hormone expert who will test your hormone levels and then prescribe the appropriate hormone dosages to re-balance them. However this is a costly option and may be beyond the financial means of many women.

An effective, safe and inexpensive alternative to reverse hair loss is to use progesterone therapy. Progesterone therapy is the self-administered use of bio-identical progesterone cream. It will achieve the following:

- Increase your progesterone level.
- Reduce your testosterone level.
- Block DHT and prevent it from causing damage.
- Enhance your blood flow to enable nutrients, needed for hair growth, to reach your hair.

34

From Perky To Sagging – Why This Has
Happened To Your Boobs

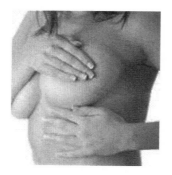

"You start out happy that you have no hips or boobs. All of a sudden you get them, and it feels sloppy. Then just when you start liking them, they start drooping."

CINDY CRAWFORD

Let me be clear from the outset. There is nothing you can do to return your breasts to the way they were in your 20s or 30s, or even early 40s.

Even breast lift surgery results are not permanent, because the breast skin and ligaments will stretch again eventually.

Sagging breasts is a natural, inevitable process that happens to all women at some point, except to women with fairly small breasts.

It is ironic that many women with small breasts dreamt of having bigger breasts when they were younger. Some may have even undergone breast augmentation procedures. But their small breasts serve them well in menopause and beyond.

Some women, who enjoyed being well endowed when they were younger, complain that during menopause their boobs are so heavy that they have to hold them up when they walk around!

The purpose of this chapter is to help you to better understand what has happened to your breasts, and why you now have sagging breasts. This may help you to free up attention that may be fixed on your sagging breasts and what has happened to them.

Breasts do not have muscle. (121) they are made of the following:

- Fat – The amount and distribution of fat determines the overall size and shape of breasts. When women are younger, their breasts have less fat and are mostly comprised of milk-producing glands.
- Milk-producing glands – They expand and shrink in response to the hormone changes that accompany different stages of the menstrual cycle and pregnancy.

They are mostly concentrated in the top outer portion of each breast, which is why this area can get tender and achy in the pre-menstrual phase. During pregnancy and before menstruation, the glands in the breast expand and become more sensitive.

After pregnancy and menopause, these glands shrink and the breast becomes mostly fat tissue in composition

- Connective tissue – Breasts are supported by ligaments (a type of connective tissue) and skin.

The connective tissue provides flexibility to the breasts. It allows the breasts to expand and then contract during the menstrual cycle and pregnancy.

Over time the skin and ligaments that support the breasts become stretched out, resulting in sagging breasts.

THE CAUSES OF SAGGING BREASTS:
A 2007 study found that there are 4 causes of sagging breasts. (122)

1. Pregnancies – The number of pregnancies is a factor in breast sagging.

During pregnancy a woman's breasts get bigger in readiness to provide milk for the newborn baby. The biggest change is in the actual composition of the breast tissue.

The milk ducts in the breast grow and branch out, almost completely replacing areas which were previously occupied by fatty tissue. The breast skin expands. After weaning, the breasts the breast size reduces but the extra skin remains.

Contrary to popular opinion, breast feeding does not contribute to sagging breasts.

2. Yo-yoing weight – Yo-yoing weight causes breast sagging. Breasts are very sensitive to weight changes.

When you gain weight, fat tends to go to your breasts first. They're also one of the first places most women lose weight from when they diet.

The thinner and heavier you get, the thinner and heavier your boobs will be, and the droopier they will be. If you keep stretching and shrinking something, it will wear out, like a sweater

3. Cigarette smoking – cigarette smoking causes breast sagging. It breaks down a protein in the skin called elastin, which gives youthful skin its elastic appearance and supports the breast.
4. Aging-

In your 20s and 30s, your boobs were their perkiest. Estrogen kept the skin and connective tissues of your breasts firm and strong.

As the years went by, the factors above contributed to a stretching of your breast skin and a deterioration of your connective tissue. The fat content of your breast increased. This made your breasts less firm.

During your 40s, breast shape continued to change. Your estrogen levels, which kept your breasts perkier in your 20s, are declining. More fat is deposited in your breasts. These factors contribute to the continuing sagging of your boobs.

Most women reach menopause (no period for 12 consecutive months) in their 50s. Menopause signals the end of a woman's reproductive years. With that comes a shutting down of the milk producing function of the breasts. The breasts not only become fattier, but they will shrink because women no longer need the milk-producing glands for breastfeeding.

You are left with breast skin that has been stretched over the years. When the tissues inside breast shrink, and the skin surrounding it doesn't, the breast looks "empty" and saggy.

35

Why Your Boobs Can Hurt Like Hell During Menopause

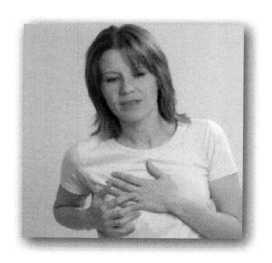

They are so sore!

"My boobs have gotten huge and they hurt like hell...
My boobs are hideously too big for me and so sore...
My boobs have hurt more than usual these past few years...
My boobs are huge and they are sore all the time. I feel like I'm nursing a whale!"

These are just a few of the comments expressed by menopausal women about their breasts.

Breast tenderness, or breast soreness or breast pain, affects up to 70% of women during their lifetime, and is most common between the ages of 30 and 50. It is a common PMS and perimenopause symptom. (124)

High levels of estrogen cause swollen and tender breasts. It increases breast size by stimulating growth of breast tissue.

While the cause of breast soreness is uncertain, it is known that high levels of estrogen causes tiny cysts to form, which are a collection of fluids that make the breasts look and feel lumpy. This may contribute to the soreness. (125)

Prior to perimenopause, breast tenderness is caused by fluctuating levels of estrogen and progesterone, during the normal menstrual cycle. In the two weeks before menstruation begins, estrogen levels are high and progesterone levels are low. This is when breast tenderness is experienced. During the next two weeks, estrogen levels fall and progesterone levels rise.

For most of the time during perimenopause, levels of estrogen are high and levels of progesterone are low. This can cause persistent breast tenderness or soreness. (126)

WHY ARE ESTROGEN LEVELS HIGH IN PERIMENOPAUSE?

The answer comes from an examination of menstrual cycles prior to perimenopause and during perimenopause.

What follows is a synopsis of the menstrual cycle prior to perimenopause:

1. The pituitary gland produces the hormone FSH (follicle stimulating hormone).
2. FSH stimulates the ovaries to develop some eggs. It also stimulates the ovaries to produce estrogen. This encourages the eggs to mature and starts to thicken the lining of the uterus so that it's ready to support a pregnancy, should fertilization occur.
3. As estrogen levels rise, which cause FSH levels to rise further to encourage an egg to mature and burst out of its sac and away from the ovary. This is called ovulation.

4. The empty sac produces large amounts of progesterone, which plays several roles in preparing the reproductive system for a potential pregnancy. As progesterone levels rise, estrogen levels fall.

As woman gets older, the numbers of eggs in her ovaries decrease. When a woman reaches perimenopause, ovulation occurs less and less frequently. There just are an insufficient number of eggs left in the ovaries to ensure that ovulation occurs every month.

The reason that estrogen levels are higher during perimenopause, than prior to it is that the body produces an increasing amount of estrogen and FSH in an attempt to develop an egg.

When ovulation does not occur, the ovaries produce just small amounts of progesterone, which is insufficient to lower the high levels of estrogen produced during the menstrual process. (127)

The end result is that during perimenopause, there are high levels of estrogen and low levels of progesterone in the body.

TREATMENTS THAT RELIEVE BREAST TENDERNESS OR SORENESS:

You must avoid traditional HRT (hormone replacement therapy). It increases your estrogen levels.

You should not use the contraceptive pill for the same reason.

To relieve breast tenderness or soreness, estrogen levels must be reduced and progesterone levels must be increased. (13)

The most effective way to do this is to get the levels of your hormones tested and then re-balanced. However this is a costly option and may be beyond the financial means of many women. There will be lab fees (hundreds of dollars) to test your hormone levels and physician fees to help you re-balance them. Often, this is not covered by health insurance policies.

A safe, effective and inexpensive way to relieve your perimenopause symptoms is to use self-administered natural progesterone cream. Natural progesterone cream will increase your progesterone level and reduce your estrogen levels.

36

Is It A Panic Attack Or A Heart Attack?

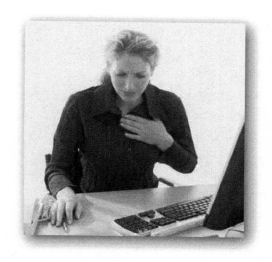

"Suddenly ... my heart started racing .... And I swear I felt it skip a beat. It felt as if my heart was going to beat right out of my chest. Then, I felt dizzy and a cold sweat broke out across my forehead. My reaction was "OMG .... I'm having a heart attack".

G. S. said that she took herself immediately to the ER, which is the right thing to do when you experience those symptoms. She was given an ECG, which revealed that her heart signs were normal and healthy.

As she had never experienced these symptoms before and as she started to notice irregularities in her period, which had been like clockwork all of her life, she wanted to know if the symptoms could be related to menopause.

I explained to her that both irregular heartbeats (racing heart, palpitations and skipped heart beats) and panic attacks are symptoms of perimenopause.

IRREGULAR HEARTBEAT AND PANIC ATTACKS
They are experienced by up to 40% of women during perimenopause.

Irregular heartbeat is more common in perimenopause than in post menopause. The heart of the average adult women beats between 60 and 100 times a minute.

A racing heart during perimenopause can have more than 200 extra heart beats per minute. (128)

Panic attack and irregular heartbeat symptoms are frighteningly similar to heart attack symptoms. (129)

Panic attack and irregular heartbeat symptoms include:

- shortness of breath
- palpitations
- chest pain
- dizziness
- vertigo
- numbness of hands and feet
- sweating
- fainting
- trembling

HEART ATTACK SYMPTOMS:
The symptoms of a heart attack are different in a woman than a man. (130)

Doctors say, in general, that the three most commonly reported symptoms when men have a heart attack are chest pain, chest discomfort, and chest pressure.

71% of women experience early warning signs of heart attack … weeks prior to their heart attack … with a sudden onset of extreme weakness and fatigue that feels like the flu – often with no chest pain at all. At the time of their heart attack, women may experience shortness of breath, weakness, and fatigue — but not always chest pressure, pain, or tightness.

Common heart attack symptoms in women include:

- As with men, a woman may experience chest pain or discomfort. But women are somewhat more likely than men to experience some of the following symptoms.
- Discomfort, tightness, uncomfortable pressure, fullness, squeezing in the center of the chest lasting more than a few minutes, or comes and goes.
- Pressure or pain that spreads to the shoulders, neck, upper back, jaw, or arms.
- Dizziness
- Nausea
- Clammy sweats
- Heart flutters
- Unexplained feelings of anxiety, fatigue or weakness – especially with exertion.
- Stomach or abdominal pain.
- Shortness of breath and difficulty breathing.

Notice how similar these symptoms are to panic attack and irregular heartbeat symptoms.

THE CAUSE OF IRREGULAR HEARTBEAT AND PANIC ATTACK SYMPTOMS DURING MENOPAUSE

They are caused by changes in the hormone levels of your body.

It is the falling estrogen levels combined with a low level of progesterone that causes irregular heartbeat and panic attack symptoms.

Panic attacks, anxiety attacks, and irregular heartbeats (as well as heart attacks) are brought about by a constriction of the blood vessels in the heart.

Estrogen has a positive effect on your blood vessels. (131) It keeps them flexible so they can relax and expand to accommodate blood flow. When estrogen levels fall, it can cause the inner chambers of the heart to contract and mimic a heart attack. This is called Cardiac Syndrome X, or Cardiac X.

Progesterone is known as your relaxing hormone. One of its functions is to keep the walls of your blood vessels relaxed, which helps to keep them dilated and prevent unnecessary constriction.

Because your body is deficient in progesterone during perimenopause, the blood vessels of your heart are more prone to constriction.

WHAT TO DO WHEN YOU EXPERIENCE ANY PANIC OR HEART SYMPTOMS FOR THE FIRST TIME

Heart attack is the number 1 killer of women, therefore, when you experience panic or heart symptoms for the first time, always suspect that it is a heart attack, and do the following:

1. Don't wait — call 911 immediately.
2. Chew, not swallow, a regular dose 325-mg aspirin. (132)
3. If necessary, have someone take you to the hospital.
4. If no other options are available, take yourself to the hospital.

More than 50% of angiograms that were done on women (an X-ray photograph of blood or lymph vessels) show no coronary disease. The most common diagnosis is cardiac syndrome X (also called cardiac X).

Cardio syndrome X patients have the symptoms of a heart attack, but an angiogram shows that there has not been a heart attack. The coronary arteries are clear of blockages. It is not life threatening and does not increase your risk of heart attack.

Cardio syndrome X is most common in menopausal women and is caused by falling estrogen and progesterone levels.

If tests show that you have not had a heart attack, your symptoms have been caused by the changing levels of estrogen and progesterone in your body. To prevent a recurrence of these symptoms, you need to re-balance the levels of estrogen and progesterone in your body.

37

Why Your # 1 Health Target Should Be A Healthy Heart

"One of the most sublime experiences we can ever have is to wake up feeling healthy after we have been sick."

RABBI HAROLD KUSHNER

Worldwide, 8.6 million women die from heart disease each year, accounting for a third of all deaths in women. 267,000 women in America die each year from heart attacks, which kill six times as many women as breast cancer.

435,000 American women have heart attacks annually; 83,000 are under age 65; 35,000 are under 55. 42% of women who have heart attacks die within 1 year, compared to 24% of men.

Research reveals that menopausal women are more frightened of breast cancer than any other illness. Yet heart disease is the number 1 killer of women. It is more deadly than all forms of cancer combined.

While 1 in 31 American women dies from breast cancer each year, 1 in 3 dies of heart disease. Yet, a national heart association survey found that only 1 in 5 American women believe that heart disease is their greatest health threat. (133)

WHY WOMEN FEAR BREAST CANCER MORE THAN HEART DISEASE?

There are 2 reasons why woman fear breast cancer more than heart disease

1. When it comes to women's health, breast cancer tends to get more attention than heart disease.

There has been effective marketing to increase awareness of breast cancer. Marketing to increase the awareness of heart disease risks has not been as effective.

- Breast cancer is a brand. A pink ribbon is an international symbol of breast cancer awareness.
- Events help to keep breast cancer in the public eye....National Breast Cancer Awareness Month, walkathons, bicycle rides etc.
- Thousands of breast cancer-themed products are developed and sold each year to keep it high in the public awareness.
- Companies advertise their products for women by associating them with the pink ribbon.

2. A diagnosis of breast cancer can knock a woman's self-confidence. Many women associate their breasts with femininity. To them, breast cancer can represent a threat of losing their breasts, and therefor losing their femininity. Removal of a breast, or both breasts, can result in a woman thinking that she is "less a woman".

MENOPAUSE INCREASES YOUR RISK OF HEART DISEASE

Studies show a woman's risk of heart disease intensifies drastically around the time of menopause, which for most women is around the age of 50.

Falling levels of estrogen during perimenopause and permanently low levels of estrogen after menopause, play a major role in the following factors conspire to significantly increase your risk of heart disease: (134)

- HDL cholesterol (good cholesterol) level will likely fall.
- LDL cholesterol (bad cholesterol) level will likely rise.
- Blood vessels will become less flexible. They do not expand and contract as they did prior to perimenopause. They become stiffer and narrower.
- Weight is likely to go up. Weight gain increases the strain on your heart

Low levels of estrogen are just one of the changes that occur in a woman's body during menopause. There are several other changes that occur in your body during menopause that greatly increases your risk of heart disease.

Researchers have found that both estrogen and progesterone have positive effects on your heart. They keep your blood vessels flexible so they can relax and expand to accommodate blood flow. (134, 135)

When your estrogen and progesterone levels are low, your blood vessels become less flexible. They do not expand and contract as they did prior to perimenopause. They become stiffer and narrower.

If your blood vessels have narrowed, your heart must work harder to push the same volume of blood through your body. This creates greater force against the blood vessel walls, putting strain on your heart. This increase in force is measured by your blood pressure.

This causes high blood pressure, also called hypertension. Hypertension is one of the biggest heart disease risk factors in menopausal women. (136)

Estrogen and progesterone also affect your cholesterol levels. Low levels of estrogen and progesterone lower HDL (good cholesterol) levels and increase LDL (bad cholesterol) levels.

HOW CHANGES IN THE LEVEL OF CORTISOL AFFECTS YOUR HEART?

Cortisol is the stress hormone. Your body produces increased amounts of cortisol when you experience stress.

High levels of cortisol curtail certain functions of your body and enhance other functions, in order to help you deal with a stressful event or situation. It ramps up your heart rate, blood pressure, and the amount of blood your heart pumps. (137)

As menopause is a time of heightened mental, emotional and physical stress for women, it can lead to chronically high cortisol levels. This leads to high blood pressure (hypertension), which is a major risk factor for heart disease.

High cortisol levels decreases the production of thyroid hormone by your body.

HOW CHANGES IN THE LEVEL OF THYROID HORMONE AFFECT YOUR HEART?

Thyroid hormone is very important for normal cardiovascular function. It, like estrogen and progesterone, helps to keep you blood vessels flexible, so they can expand and contract according to the flow of blood through them.

26% of menopausal women have an underactive thyroid condition … known as hypothyroidism. It is a condition in which there is insufficient thyroid hormone levels to efficiently manage the metabolism … inclusive of the heart function.

When there is not enough thyroid hormone, neither the heart nor the blood vessels can function normally. (138)

In hypothyroidism the heart muscle becomes weakened, and can no longer pump as vigorously as it should. In addition, the heart muscle cannot fully relax in between heart beats. It causes blood vessels to stiffen, which produces hypertension.

Hypothyroidism increases the level of insulin in your body.

HOW CHANGES IN THE LEVEL OF INSULIN AFFECT YOUR HEART?

Falling and low levels of estrogen are associated with high levels of insulin in the body. Estrogen enables insulin to regulate your blood sugar level. Low levels of estrogen are associated with insulin resistance, which causes diabetes.

Almost all menopausal women have insulin resistance to some degree.

Diabetes itself significantly raises the risk of heart disease. Women with diabetes have it worse, on average, than men with diabetes. The risk for heart disease is six times higher for women with diabetes than those without. (139)

High levels of insulin increase the risk of heart disease because of the following:

- It raises the level of LDL cholesterol (bad cholesterol) in the blood, while lowering the level of HDL cholesterol (good cholesterol).
- It promotes the formation of dangerous plaques that clogs arteries.
- Excessive insulin boosts inflammation throughout the body, including within the lining of blood vessels. Inflammation of blood vessels is associated with heart disease.

In order to reduce your risk of heart disease, it goes without saying that you should do the following:

1. Eat properly and on time as discussed previously.
2. Increase you activity level. You should do a form of aerobic activity every day.
3. Engage with a stress reduction technique regularly.
4. Address balancing estrogen and progesterone levels.

These activities will help to regulate the levels of cortisol, thyroid, insulin, progesterone and estrogen in your body, helping to minimize the risk of a heart disease as a menopause woman.

38

Menopause And Arthritis – The Kissing Cousins

"Knee pain troubles me more than any other menopause symptom!"

J. M.

Do you suffer from the following?

- Wake in the morning with knees or/and hips or/and hands or/and feet that are stiff and achy?
- Feel stiffness and pain in your joints when you get up from a seated position?

Although joint pains are not THE most common menopause symptom that distinction goes to hot flashes it bothers woman more than any other symptom.

A recent midlife population survey found that, more women reported joint pains and aches, as the symptom that bothers them more than any other symptom. (140)

41% of women pre menopause, and 57% of women two years post menopause, report that they experience significant joint pains and aches.

IS JOINT PAIN ARTHRITIS?

Yes it is. Joint pain is caused by inflammation. Arthritis is inflammation of one or more joints. (141) Also, the derivation of the word arthritis provides us with a clue to the answer. It comes from the Greek "Arthron" meaning joint and the Latin "itis" meaning inflammation.

There are more than 100 forms of Arthritis. The most common form is osteoarthritis, often called "wear and tear" arthritis. Osteoarthritis is a condition in which there is wear and tear of the protective covering around the bones that form the joints. As a result, the bones rub together causing pain, swelling, and loss of motion of the joints.

DOES MENOPAUSE CAUSE ARTHRITIS?

The North American Menopause Society says that it is unclear whether menopause is the cause of arthritis or if it is aging or if it is a combination of both. However they do say that it is clear that after menopause there is an increase in the severity and frequency of arthritic symptoms.

It is also clear that the time when most women begin to experience joint pains, coincides with the time they experience menopause symptoms. The onset of arthritis is gradual and usually begins after the age of 40. (142)

More women get arthritis than men. 60% of the sufferers are women. It is estimated that the majority of women have it by age 65 and that 80 percent of women over 75 years of age have it. (143)

WHAT IS THE LINK BETWEEN MENOPAUSE AND ARTHRITIS?

It is falling levels of estrogen during perimenopause and low levels of estrogen after menopause. Post menopause estrogen levels are 10% of what they are prior to perimenopause.

The research linking estrogen depletion to joint pain is as follows

- In 2005 two noted researchers, David T. Felson, M.D., of Boston University Clinical Epidemiology Unit, and Steven R. Cummings,

M.D., of California Pacific Medical Center Research Institute and University of California, San Francisco, concluded that there is a link between estrogen deprivation and joint pain. (144)

- A study conducted in 2010 found that reduced levels of estrogen causes menopause joint pain. (145)
- A case study from a medical doctor (146)

Joyce is a 52 years old, post-menopausal typist who came to see me in the office because of joint pain in her hands which keeps her up at night with aching, and interferes with her job as a typist. She was fine until about three years ago when she went into menopause and stopped her menstrual cycles.

I explained to Joyce that she had fairly classical Menopausal Arthritis caused by an inflammatory response associated with declining estrogen levels. I have noted this in many of my patients. The inflammatory process is usually relieved by bio-identical estrogen as a topical cream. Joyce's lab panel showed low estrogen levels, and Joyce was started on her bio-identical hormone program. Six weeks later, Joyce reports complete relief of symptoms. Her arthritis pains have gone. In addition, Joyce reports that she went off the bio-identical hormone cream for a week to see what would happen, and sure enough, the arthritis came back, only to be relieved again by resuming the hormone cream. This is a fairly typical story that I have seen over and over again.

WHAT YOU CAN DO TO RELIEVE MENOPAUSE JOINT PAIN?

1. Include a stress reduction technique in your life. Do yoga or meditation, or some other stress reduction technique, regularly.

Physical pain causes stress. Your body increases its production of cortisol – the stress hormone – during times of stress. Cortisol acts as an inflammatory agent.

Sustained stress (the kind that you experience with joint pain) can cause inflammation to spread at a rapid rate

2. Consider estrogen therapy to increase you estrogen levels. It helps to relieve joint pains.

Conventional medicine practitioners may prescribe synthetic estrogen therapy to treat joint pain, in the form of a pill or cream.

The pill taken orally enters the blood stream. It increases your risk of breast cancer and blood clots.

The cream can be applied to your joints. It carries a lower risk of breast cancer, because it is localized. It doesn't enter your blood stream.

Physicians who practice integrative medicine are more likely to favor natural bioidentical estrogen therapy .... Taken as a cream that is applied locally to your joints. It does not bear the health risks associated with synthetic estrogen therapy.

3. Engage in a daily aerobic exercise.
4. If possible, increase the strength of the muscles around the joint.

I would be surprised if you don't react to this by saying something like "You must be joking. Exercise is the last thing that I want to do ... with the way I feel".

Here is what the Mayo Clinic says about exercise and joint pain:

"Though you might think exercise will aggravate your joint pain and stiffness, that's not the case. Lack of exercise actually can make your joints even more painful and stiff. That's because keeping your muscles and surrounding tissue strong is crucial to maintaining support for your bones. Not exercising weakens those supporting muscles, creating more stress on your joints." (147)

5. Eliminate all processed food from your diet. They contain sugar, which exacerbates inflammation.

Increase intake of non-processed food such as: meat, fish, milk, eggs, legumes, fruits, grains and vegetables.

Make a special effort to include foods rich in omega 3 fatty acids. They decrease the level of inflammation around your joints.

Two foods that are richest in omega 3 fatty acids are flaxseed and walnuts. Fish is a rich source of it as well, especially salmon, herring, mackerel, sardines, halibut, scallops, shrimp, and rainbow trout.

6. If you are not averse to taking supplements, there are 2 supplements that have helped many women to relieve joint aches and pains....glucosamine sulfate and methylsulfonylmethane, or MSM. Glucosamine relieves pain and heals joints by building up the cartilage that protects the ends of bones. MSM reduces the inflammatory chemicals called cytokines that causes joint aches and pains during menopause.

39

Women Don't Fart ... Except Maybe Sometimes During Menopause

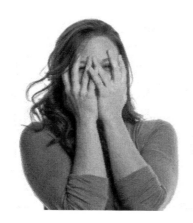

HAVE YOU BEEN FARTING MORE SINCE THE ONSET OF
MENOPAUSE?

Farting is part of the universal human experience. Farting knows no borders: every person from every corner of the globe breaks wind. (The average person toots 14 times per day, in case you were wondering.)

There have been more than 150 terms used to describe a fart. Some of the more descriptive references include air biscuit, anal applause, breaking wind, passing wind, sphincter whistle, and floater.

The world's oldest recorded joke from 1900 B.C. is about; you guessed it, ancient air biscuits. (148)

Throughout history, the chance to make an occasional fart joke has often proven irresistible, even to such influential authors as Chaucer, Shakespeare, and Mark Twain. There are references to farting in the following:

- Dante's The Inferno (14th Century)
- Chaucer's The Canterbury Tales (14th Century)
- William Shakespeare's A Comedy of Errors (1594)
- Mark Twain's 1601 (1880)
- James Joyce's Ulysses (1922)

WHAT IS A FART ANYWAY?
When you eat, you don't swallow just your food. You also swallow air, which contains gases like nitrogen and oxygen. Small amounts of these gases travel through your digestive system as you digest your food.

When you digest food, gas is released in the form of hydrogen, methane and carbon dioxide. As the gas builds up, your body needs to get rid of it – this is done by either burping (belching) or flatulence (farting).

Farts make a sound when they escape due to the vibrations of your rectum. The loudness may vary depending on how much pressure is behind the gas, as well as the tightness of your sphincter muscles.

WHAT DOES FARTING HAVE TO DO WITH MENOPAUSE?
Two-thirds of women report that they experience increased stomach gas during menopause, according to a survey conducted by the Market Research Institute. (149) When asked which menopause symptoms they experienced the most, the following were the results:

- Gas was 69%
- Hot flashes was 66%
- Disturbed sleep was 65%
- Mood swings was 64%

An increase in stomach gas during menopause leads to an increase of farting.

Strictly speaking, the increase in stomach gas occurs during perimenopause. It is caused by changes in the levels of estrogen and progesterone from their levels prior to perimenopause.

During perimenopause estrogen levels fluctuate. This means that it rises and falls periodically. Progesterone falls continuously during perimenopause.

Fluctuating estrogen levels and falling progesterone causes your digestive system to produce more gas during perimenopause, than prior to it. Your body normally produces some gas during the digestive process throughout your life. It increases during perimenopause because the balance of the bacteria involved in the digestive process is disturbed by the changing levels of estrogen and progesterone.

Your intestines contain "good bacteria" and "bad bacteria". Both are necessary for optimal digestion. (150) When the good and bad bacteria are in balance, healthy digestion occurs. When the balance between good and bad bacteria is upset (an increase in bad bacteria), the digestive patterns of the body are altered, resulting in an increase in the production of gas during menopause.

HOW TO RELIEVE EXCESS STOMACH GAS DURING MENOPAUSE?

As excess stomach gas is caused by changing levels of estrogen and progesterone during perimenopause, which causes imbalance between them, the most effective way to relieve it is to re-balance the levels of estrogen and progesterone in your body.

However many women are averse to hormone therapy. If you are averse to hormone therapy, here are some tips that will help you to reduce stomach gas during menopause

- Change your eating habits – Eating big portions can lower digestive function, and so it is best to eat smaller portions more frequently.

Eat a smaller breakfast, lunch and supper than you have been accustomed to eating and eat a healthy snack (fruit, nuts, yoghurt etc.) between those meals and after supper.

Chew your food more slowly. This will break your food into smaller chunks and allows the digestive enzymes in your saliva to do their work. It will reduce gas production in your body

- Change your diet – Certain foods tend to cause a build-up of gas, so consumption of them should be reduced. These include beans, broccoli, onions, beets, Brussel sprouts, cabbage, lentils, breakfast cereals, whole wheat flour and other some other foods that are generally regarded to be healthy foods. It is advisable to develop a complete list of foods that tend to produce gas and minimize your intake of them.

It is ironic that many of these foods are recommended by The North American Menopause Society to help women reduce their menopause symptoms, and yet they cause your body to increase the production of gas during menopause.

Make no mistake though …. These foods ARE effective at reducing many of the symptoms of menopause

- Exercise regularly – Exercise increases the flow of blood through your body. This stimulates the digestive system and helps it work more efficiently.

Increased gas during menopause is more prevalent in women who lead sedentary lifestyles. Being more active prevents it. It stimulates your digestive system

- There is a natural product that helps to prevent the build-up of gas in the digestive process. It is called Beano.

Beano contains a natural food enzyme that helps prevent gas before it starts. It works with your body's digestion to break down the complex carbohydrates in gassy foods, like fresh vegetables, whole grain breads and beans, making them more digestible. Beano enables you to enjoy your favorite healthy foods, whether at home, in a restaurant or at a friend's house, without worrying about gas. Beano is not a drug.

Beano contains an enzyme from a natural source that works with your body's digestion. It breaks down the complex carbohydrates found in gassy foods into simpler, easily digestible sugars before they reach the colon, preventing gas before it starts.

40

Are fibroids making your life a living hell?

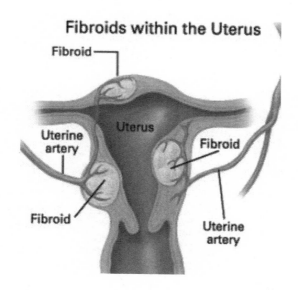

Fibroids within the Uterus

Fibroid

Uterus

Uterine artery

Fibroid

Fibroid

Uterine artery

Do you have fibroid that causes heavy painful periods?
Do you have Flooding painful periods?
Do you know all of treatment options for fibroids?

If you are 50 years old, there is at least a 70% chance that you have one or more fibroids. (151). Fibroids are growths on the uterus. They are not life threatening. They are almost always benign (not cancerous). Rarely (less than one in 1,000) a cancerous fibroid will occur.

A minuscule percentage of women experience extreme pain or discomfort from a fibroid. This occurs when a fibroid grows extremely large, creating pressure on nearby organs. A fibroid can be as small as an apple seed or as big as a grapefruit.

Abnormal uterine bleeding is the most common symptom of a fibroid. (152) Symptoms include the following:

1. Bleeding between periods.
2. Heavy bleeding during your period, sometimes with blood clots.
3. Periods that may last longer than normal.
4. Needing to urinate more often.
5. Pelvic cramping or pain with periods.
6. Feeling fullness or pressure in your lower belly.
7. Pain during intercourse.

They are most common in women who are in their 40s and early 50s.

ESTROGEN DOMINANCE

No one knows exactly what causes them. However there is a link between their development and the levels of estrogen and progesterone in a woman's body, due to the estrogen dominance, where estrogen levels are high relative to the level of progesterone.

Stress plays a significant role in the growth of fibroids, by increasing the dominance of estrogen. When you experience stress, your body decreases its production of progesterone. (153)

STRESS DURING MENOPAUSE

Many women say that menopause is the most stressful phase of their lives, especially women who are experiencing moderate to severe menopause symptoms.

Estrogen dominance triggers changes in the ratios and levels of all the other hormones in your body, including the major hormones insulin, cortisol and thyroid. It leads to erratic production of these hormones by your body.

Collectively, estrogen, progesterone, insulin, cortisol and thyroid hormones control and affect all of the systems of your body. The changes in the ratios and levels of these hormones disturb all the systems of your body, which is the cause of all of your menopause symptoms. When those symptoms are moderate to severe, they cause you to experience mental, emotional and physical stress.

TREATMENT OF FIBROIDS

Most fibroids shrink to the point of irrelevance after menopause. However until you reach menopause (final menstrual period), you may be concerned about managing the size of your fibroids.

While there are several treatment options available to women with fibroids, too many doctors recommend just one treatment, Hysterectomy. They do not inform women of the other options available to them, or the consequences of this invasive surgery.

Every year approximately 600,000 hysterectomies are performed in the US. Up to 50% of the hysterectomies are done to treat fibroids...a benign condition... according to the National Uterine Foundation (154). More hysterectomies are done because of fibroids, than any other problem of the uterus.

10% of hysterectomies are performed because of an existing cancer condition. Critics of rampant hysterectomies agree that a hysterectomy is necessary when cancer is present.

Critics of rampant hysterectomies say that woman who have an extremely large fibroid (i.e. – the size of a grapefruit), that causes severe pain, are also legitimate candidates for hysterectomies. However these represent a very small percentage of the hysterectomies performed.

A panel convened by the American College of Obstetricians and Gynecologists found that 76% of all hysterectomies performed today do not meet the criteria for this surgery (155). They are being done unnecessarily. Dr Ernst Bartsich, MD, and associate professor of obstetrics and gynecology at the New York Hospital-Cornell Medical Center in New York said:

"I believe many women are conceding to a hysterectomy for fibroid tumors because they are led to believe it's the only solution — and that is wrong!"

WHAT TO DO, IF YOU HAVE BEEN DIAGNOSED WITH FIBROIDS?

1. Consider all of the fibroid treatment options. (156) Discuss them with your healthcare provider and family and friends.
2. As fibroid growth is associated with too much estrogen in your body and not enough progesterone, consider re-balancing your hormones. Not only will this reduce a fibroid, but it will also relieve many of your menopause symptoms.
3. As stress is a significant factor in fibroid growth, consider doing one or more stress reduction techniques, mentioned previously, regularly.

41

Has Menopause Left You Feeling Dry? ...
No I Don't Mean "Down There"

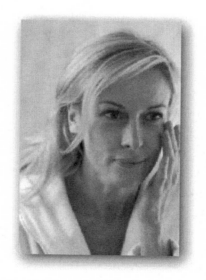

"I never associated my eye problems with menopause"

M. T.

D o you ever experience the following?

- Eye fatigue after short periods of reading.
- Blurred vision, often worsening at the end of the day or after focusing for a prolonged period.

- A dry or gritty sensation in the eye.
- Eye irritation.
- Eye itching.
- A burning sensation in your eyes.
- Sore eyes.
- Red eyes.
- Periods of excessive tearing.

These are symptoms of Dry Eye Syndrome, often referred to simply as dry eyes or dry eye.

Dry eyes are a little known symptom of menopause experienced by approximately 61 percent of menopausal women, according to the Society for Women's Health Research. Yet only 16 per cent of women associate their dry eye symptoms with menopause, according to a survey of menopausal women with dry eye symptoms.

For years, it has been recognized that dry eye is one of the leading causes of patient visits to ophthalmologists. It is estimated that over 10 million people in the United States have this problem. It occurs predominantly in middle age women, and much less frequently in men.

As the condition is so prevalent in women of menopausal age, and not in younger women and not in men, the link between dry eyes and menopause will be discussed.

WHAT IS DRY EYE SYNDROME?

To understand dry eye, you need to know a bit about the anatomy of your eyes.

To help keep your eyes comfortable and vision optimal, a thin film of tears coats the eyes. This film consists of 3 layers:

- An underlying gel composed of mucous – it helps the overlying watery layer to spread evenly over your eyes
- A middle watery layer that consists of a salt solution – it keeps your eyes moist and comfortable, as well as to help flush out any dust, debris, or foreign objects that may get into your eyes

- An overlying layer that is oily (like the oils on your skin) – its function is to help decrease evaporation of the watery layer beneath it

Dry eyes occur when one of these layers of the tear film is missing or deficient.

There are two types of dry eyes (157) … water-deficient and evaporative.

Water-deficient dry eye is due to a lack of watery substance in the middle layer. Evaporative dry eyes are due to lack of oil in the overlying layer to prevent evaporation of the watery substance in the middle layer. Water-deficient dry eyes are the more common.

THE LINKS BETWEEN DRY EYES AND MENOPAUSE

Dryness is a common complaint during menopause. Your hair, skin and "down there" seem to experience it. They seem to need a bit more attention (and lubrication) than when you were younger. And, so do your eyes.

There are 2 links between dry eyes and menopause:

- Changing hormone levels during menopause
- Loss of collagen in your body during menopause

CHANGING HORMONE LEVELS DURING MENOPAUSE

You are probably aware that all of your menopause symptoms are caused by changing hormone levels during menopause. Almost all of your symptoms are associated with changing levels of estrogen, but not this one. Researchers have found that dry eyes are associated with falling androgen levels. (158) The best known and predominant androgen is testosterone.

During perimenopause your androgen level falls. In post menopause the level of androgens in your body is considerably lower than it was prior to perimenopause.

Androgens regulate the production of the salty solution of the watery middle layer of your tear film and the outer oily layer of the tear film. During menopause, lower levels of testosterone causes a lack of the salty solution and protective oil in the tear film (160), which brings about dry eyes.

LOSS OF COLLAGEN AND DRY EYES

There have been no studies to examine the link between loss of collagen and dry eyes. However, it is inconceivable that the loss of collagen in your body during menopause does not contribute to dry eyes.

Collagen is the most abundant protein in your body. It is the main connective tissue that holds you together. It is a vital component of most structures in your body. (160)

Your eyes are made up of 80% collagen. The tissues in the glands that produce the salty solution and the oil for your tear film are made of collagen.

During menopause the level of collagen in your body decreases significantly. It follows the decrease of estrogen in your body during menopause.

Science has long known that estrogen plays a vital role in maintaining the level of collagen in your body. (161) The level of collagen in your body follows the same pattern as the level of estrogen, as you age. Falling estrogen levels = falling collagen levels.

Falling levels of collagen in your body weakens and degrades the tissues of your body, including the tissues in your eyes.

HOW TO ELIMINATE DRY EYE SYMPTOMS?

Research conducted by a professor of ophthalmology at Harvard Medical School found that testosterone cream is a safe and effective therapy for the treatment of dry eye. (162)

You may also want to consider bio-identical estriol therapy to increase the level of collagen in your body (and eyes). A review of 45 scientific studies found estriol to be an effective and safe treatment that increases the level of collagen in the body. (163) Estriol is the weakest of the three estrogens in your body (the other estrogens are estradiol and estrone). Estriol does not have any of the health risks associated with taking estradiol.

If you decide to use estriol to raise the level of collagen in your body, it is advisable to supplement it by also using natural bio-identical progesterone cream. Your progesterone level falls continuously during perimenopause.

In post menopause, your body still makes a little estrogen, but it makes no progesterone.

Progesterone will ensure that estrogen is received and used by the cells of your body. Progesterone helps make estrogen receptors more sensitive. An estrogen receptor is a molecule in a cell that makes the cell sensitive to receiving estrogen.

42

Have You Been Taking More From Alcohol ...
Or Is It Taking More From You?

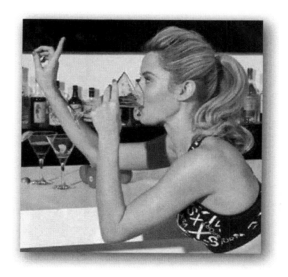

"One more drink and I'll be under the host."

MAE WEST

"Menopause really isn't that bad!"

Well, maybe some women who experience just mild menopause symptoms will say that menopause isn't that bad. However just ask any of the millions of menopausal woman who experience moderate to severe symptoms …. And you will get an entirely different response.

Here is a small selection of what women have said in response to the question "what has menopause been like for you?"

"I went from eternally optimistic happy go lucky hippie chick to suicidal demonic vampires in a day, and stayed there for 18 months."

"This has been the worst 4 yrs. of my life …I can't sleep. I can't think straight… hot flashes that seem to never end day and night…night sweats are horrible….and my moods are out of this world."

"I'm bleeding like a slaughtered pig, running out of sanitary products, feel sick, been up all night, can't sleep with my husband so am in spare room, forgot to get things out of the freezer for dinner, lost my glasses, and my legs are so painful it hurts to walk."

"The hot flashes weren't too bad at first. But now they've become unbearable. I feel like I'm locked in a sauna. I get dizzy and sweat profusely, I feel sick to my stomach and I have been having 4 or more an hour and I can't stand it anymore."

"I've been putting up with this debilitating thing for the last 5 years and it's not getting any better. I am depressed. I have aches and joint pain, headaches, insomnia, mood swings, terrible weight gain, memory loss, and anger. I wake up sweating and panicking"

"My life as I knew it has changed forever… I feel like I lost my sanity and made decisions that were life altering. Physically, I went from being very energetic and physically fit and trim, to overweight, fatigued, pain all over and a hot sweaty MESS! What should be the best years of my life are now being wasted in this dark world we call menopause."

"I feel like a hot mess more than I feel normal…whatever that is any more. My hair is falling out, my skin is a mess, I've gained 15 lbs. and can't get it off and the emotions and sense of no control suck! I am 44 and still have young kids…..this has been very challenging and life altering."

"I'm having migraine headaches way too often, more than I ever have before. I feel I'm falling apart mentally and physically. I have rolling hot flashes now followed by sweats and chills. And I'm an emotional basket case."

"It's like aliens have invaded my body and I have no control. The exhaustion, joint pain, racing thoughts when trying to sleep is hell on earth. So tired, I either want to cry or sleep."

Is it any wonder that menopausal women can be tempted by alcohol to escape their misery ... if even for just a brief time?

But this is a bad idea. Alcohol worsens hot flashes, night sweats and mental and emotional symptoms.

HOW YOUR BODY RESPONDS TO ALCOHOL INTAKE?

Once alcohol is in your system, your body makes metabolizing it a priority. That means that it will stop metabolizing anything else in order to first get the alcohol metabolized. (164)

The reason for this is because unlike protein, carbohydrates, and fat, there is nowhere for alcohol to be stored in our body so it has be metabolized first.

When you consume an alcoholic drink, the alcohol moves directly into the bloodstream without being metabolized in the stomach. It only takes five minutes for alcohol to become detectable in the bloodstream, where it then travels to the liver to be metabolized.

For most people it takes about two hours for the liver to metabolize a single drink. If you continue to drink alcohol faster than your liver can metabolize it, the excess alcohol is carried by the bloodstream to the brain and other areas of the body.

Studies have shown that alcohol interferes with the body processes that maintain healthy blood glucose levels. Alcohol makes your body less responsive to insulin. (165) When your body becomes less responsive to insulin, it increases insulin production in an attempt to regulate blood sugar levels.

Alcohol consumption also increases the level of cortisol in your body and it disturbs the performance of your thyroid hormone, which regulates your metabolism.

Whenever the healthy functioning of your insulin, cortisol and thyroid is disturbed, you can expect your menopause symptoms to worsen.

HOW ALCOHOL INTAKE WORSENS HOT FLASHES?

Alcohol causes vasodilation, or the widening of blood vessels. Your heart rate and blood pressure increase, and your blood vessels open wide to allow more rapid blood flow. This creates heat and redness.

Also, a higher level of insulin in your body brings about more hot flashes and night sweats:

1. Your body temperature is controlled by the hypothalamus … a part of your brain.
2. Your hypothalamus tries to maintain your core body temperature within a comfortable "thermoneutral zone". (166)
3. When your core temperature rises above the zone's upper threshold, you sweat; when it drops below the lower threshold, you shiver.
4. Insulin raises your core body temperature. (167)
5. Your hypothalamus responds by inducing a hot flash/night sweat to cool your body.

HOW ALCOHOL INTAKE WORSENS EMOTIONAL AND MENTAL SYMPTOMS?

Alcohol causes your insulin and cortisol levels to rise. High cortisol levels decreases the production of thyroid hormone by your body.

The collective changes in the levels of these 3 hormones create imbalances in the neurotransmitters serotonin, dopamine, GABA, and other neurotransmitters as well.

Neurotransmitters are chemical messengers that transmit thought from one cell to the next, allowing your brain cells to "talk to each other". They control all of your mental and emotional responses. (168)

The neurotransmitters are further affected by alcohol itself. As alcohol reaches the brain in minutes after it is consumed, it alters the levels of these neurotransmitters.

The changes in the levels of these neurotransmitters cause all of the emotional and mental menopause symptoms.

WHAT SHOULD YOU DO ABOUT YOUR ALCOHOL INTAKE?
It is a matter of personal preference.

However, now that you are more informed of the consequences of alcoholic intake during menopause, it would be advisable to restrict your intake of alcohol to no more than one drink per day … when your symptoms are mild to moderate. When they are severe, it would advisable to abstain from it.

43

Do You Have A Problem With Caffeine ... Or A Problem Without Caffeine?

"As long as there was coffee in the world, how bad could things be?"

CASSANDRA CLARE

"Every morning I long to hold you ... I need you, I want you, I have to have you ... your warmth, your smell, your taste.."

Could this be you speaking?
It is estimated that ninety percent of Americans, including kids consume caffeine every day. It is everywhere. It's in:

1. Coffee
2. Tea
3. Sodas like Coke and Pepsi and others
4. Chocolate
5. products containing chocolate or cocoa like cakes, donuts, cookies, ice cream, candy, and cereals
6. power and energy drinks

You were introduced to caffeine as a child. It has an association with pleasure and it has an addictive quality.

If you have been trying to reduce your intake of caffeine and are finding it hard to do, it is not surprising.

WHAT HAPPENS IN YOUR BODY WHEN YOU CONSUME FOOD OR DRINK CONTAINING CAFFEINE?

Caffeine passes directly into your bloodstream through your stomach and travels first to the brain, where it causes effects in as little as 15 minutes. (169)

Caffeine increases activity in your brain cells. Your body senses this increased activity and interprets it as a threat. It automatically increases production of cortisol and adrenaline (fight or flight response) to help you deal with what it perceives as a threat. As a result:

- Your pupils dilate.
- Your airway opens up.
- Your heart beats faster.
- Your blood vessels on the surface constrict to slow blood flow from cuts and increase blood flow to muscles.
- Your blood pressure rises.
- Your blood flow to the stomach slows.
- Your liver releases sugar into the bloodstream for extra energy.

The end result is a temporary increase in mental alertness and thought processing, while reducing drowsiness and fatigue.

Caffeine continues to affect your brain as long as it remains in your blood. The average half-life of caffeine in the adult bloodstream is about 6 hours.

This means that it takes this long for its concentration in your bloodstream to reduce by half. If you have 200 mg of coffee at mid-day, you would still have 100mg in your blood at around 6 PM.

When the caffeine rush is over and adrenaline levels drop ... fatigue, irritability, inability to concentrate, headache and weariness take over, setting the stage for a big caffeine — and sugar craving.

WHY YOU SHOULD RESTRICT YOUR INTAKE OF CAFFEINE DURING MENOPAUSE?

As the dose of caffeine in your body gets higher and then wanes, it causes spikes and dips in the levels of the neurotransmitters in your brain, which regulate your emotions.

It also causes fluctuations in the levels of hormones that regulate other parts of your body. These changes increase the frequency and severity of the following menopause symptoms:

- Hot flashes and night sweats
- Mood swings
- Anxiety
- Depression
- Irritability
- Panic attacks
- Irregular heartbeat
- Insomnia
- Frequent urination
- Fatigue
- Headaches

Caffeine disturbs the levels of 3 major hormones in your body ... insulin, cortisol and thyroid hormone. As your body operates as a holistic system, its parts are interconnected.

A change in their levels disturbs the levels of all of the hormones in your body. This will worsen your entire menopause symptoms ... not just the symptoms noted above.

HOT FLASHES/NIGHT SWEATS AND CAFFEINE

A recent study of menopausal women found that caffeine triggers an increase in hot flashes and night sweats in postmenopausal women. Over 1800 women were studied. Nearly 85% of them said they consume caffeine through tea, coffee, or soda. (170)

Other researchers have found that caffeine worsens hot flashes and night sweats in premenopausal woman as well. Caffeine reduces the effectiveness of insulin. (171)

This means that your body needs to produce more insulin than is normally needed, whenever you consume food.

As mentioned previously, higher levels of insulin in your body bring about more hot flashes and night sweats, via the "thermoneutral zone" and the hypothalamus response.

HOW CAFFEINE WORSENS THE OTHER SYMPTOMS?

Caffeine causes your insulin and cortisol levels to rise. High cortisol levels decreases the production of thyroid hormone by your body, collectively create imbalances in the neurotransmitters serotonin, dopamine and GABA, which cause all of the emotional and mental menopause symptoms mentioned above.

WHAT SHOULD YOU DO ABOUT YOUR CAFFEINE INTAKE?

Like alcohol intake decision, yes or no to caffeine, is a matter of personal preference.

I know that if my menopause symptoms were affecting the quality of my life, I would greatly restrict my intake of foods and drinks containing caffeine.

I am a coffee lover. I would not give it up. However, after my morning cup of coffee, I would have no more coffee for the rest of the day.

I would certainly eliminate sodas like Coke and Pepsi, which are laden with added sugars as well as caffeine.

44

The Sugar Monster Lurking Within You ....
And Menopause

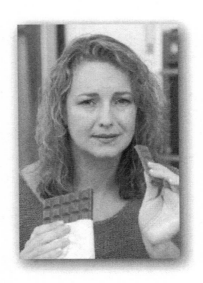

"There is nothing better than a friend, unless it is a friend with chocolate."

LINDA GRAYSON

Sugar cravings can instigate one of the most insidious downward spirals in a menopausal woman.

It can happen fast. One minute, you're indulging in a small piece of chocolate; the next, you've devoured the entire box of chocolates. You may feel awful as a result, but you are still craving more.

If you eat something high in refined sugar, your blood sugar level sky-rockets... and then crashes. Your brain interprets that crash as the need for more of that fast-acting sugar, that mid-afternoon craving for chocolate. So you eat something sugary to silence the craving and you get another spike, a dip, a spike, and then a dip again.

This is how your body responds when you satisfy your sugar craving:

1. You eat food or consume a drink high in refined sugar.
2. Refined sugar causes your blood sugar level to soar.
3. Your body responds to the high level of blood sugar (which is also called glucose), by increasing the levels of insulin in your body to a commensurate level.
4. Insulin takes the glucose from your blood and provides it to the cells of your body for energy, thus depleting the level of glucose in your blood.
5. Around 2 hours later you experience low blood sugar symptoms ..... Such as weakness, tiredness, drowsiness, dizziness, irritability and hunger.
6. You crave sugar again as a result of the low-blood-sugar condition ... and so the cycle repeats itself.

Not only does your blood sugar go up and down when you consume food or drink that is high in refined sugar, but the level of insulin in your body goes up and down as well.

Your body operates as a holistic system .... Its parts are interconnected. A change in the level of insulin gives rise to changing levels of other hormones, like cortisol and thyroid hormone. This in turn sets off changes to the levels of still other hormones.

The roller coaster rises and falls in the level of insulin in your body, in response to your intake of refined sugar, causes an imbalance in all the hormones in your body. This causes worsening menopause symptoms.

MENOPAUSE SYMPTOMS THAT ARE WORSENED WHEN YOU EAT REFINED SUGAR

Every menopause symptom is affected by your intake of refined sugar, because or the hormonal disturbance it causes. However refined sugar intake has a bigger impact on some symptoms, than others. Here are the symptoms most affected when you consume refined sugar:

- Hot flashes/night sweats
- Mood swings
- Depression
- Anxiety
- Panic attacks
- Irritability
- Irregular heartbeat
- Fatigue
- Weight gain
- Impaired concentration and memory
- Insomnia

Most of these symptoms can be categorized as mental and emotional responses to your intake of sugar.

Those symptoms not falling under the umbrella of mental and emotional responses are hot flashes/night sweats and weight gain. Insomnia is caused by the mental and emotional symptoms and hot flashes/night sweats.

Much has already been written about the effect that refined sugar has on weight gain. I will not discuss this in this post.

What follows is a synopsis of the effects of refined sugar on hot flashes/ night sweats and on mental and emotional symptoms.

EFFECTS THAT REFINED SUGAR HAS ON HOT FLASHES/NIGHT SEATS

As already covered, when you eat refined sugar your blood sugar level soars and your body responds by increasing the level of insulin in your body. Insulin raises your core body temperature. Your hypothalamus responds by inducing a hot flash/night sweat to cool your body.

EFFECTS THAT REFINED SUGAR HAS ON YOUR EMOTIONAL AND MENTAL RESPONSES

Your emotional and mental condition is regulated by your brain.

Glucose is the fuel on which your brain operates. For your brain to function optimally, it requires a steady supply of glucose. (172) Your brain does not store glucose, as other parts of your body do. It gets it from your blood.

When you consume refined sugar, your blood sugar soars. This would seem good for your brain, as it receives an abundant supply of the fuel it needs. However, as already covered, soaring blood sugar causes your body to increase production of insulin. Insulin removes glucose from your blood and stores it in the cells of your body, thus depriving your brain of blood sugar.

Soaring and crashing blood sugar levels caused by the intake of refined sugar affects the levels and performance of the neurotransmitters in your brain, regulating all of your emotional and mental responses.

Try to keep your process sugar intake to a minimum possible. A general recommendation would be to try and keep your sugar intake to equal or less than 10 grams of sugars per serving. That would minimize the effects of sugars on menopause symptoms.

Also, increase your sugar intake that derives from natural sugar products such as fruits and vegetables. It would help to replace the process sugar craving, regulate blood glucose and reduce production of insulin, thus, reduce the frequency and the severity of the menopause symptoms.

45

Coping With Menopause At Work

"The first indication of menopause is a broken thermo-stat. It's either that or your weight...God; middle age is an unending insult."

DOROTHEA BENTON FRANK

Several patients have expressed their concerns to me about the effects that menopause is having on their work.

One woman's struggle with menopause at work explained that she works in a male dominated environment and the majority of people are younger men and younger women.

She said that she feels that it would be inappropriate for her to talk about menopause to her boss or colleagues at work, and yet her menopause symptoms are having a negative effect on her performance at work.

She told me about one recent incident. During a meeting with a client, she said that she came across as muddled. At one point she mispronounced the client's name and at another point she used a different client's name, when referring to this client.

She told me that she had been experiencing disturbed sleep for several nights and it embarrassed about what had happened and that her confidence was plummeting.

Another patient of mine explained that she would be overcome with tears at inappropriate moments at work, with mood swings and sudden memory blanks.

Her hot flashes were obvious and clearly visible. As she had seen women at work being teased when they were having hot flashes, she was concerned about becoming a figure of fun to some of her colleagues.

She said that her colleagues and bosses had noticed the changes in her and some of them even commented to her about it. She was concerned about her next appraisal, and how the symptoms of menopause could affect her career. She said that her professional self-esteem hit the floor.

She said that she never expected that menopause could cause her professional life to fall apart.

MENOPAUSE AT WORK

Talking about menopause is still regarded as taboo in parts of our society. Talking about menopause at work is possibly more so than elsewhere in society. It is not regarded in the same light as pregnancy and childbirth in most companies.

How women are coping with menopause at work is a topic that needs much more attention than it gets.

How to deal with menopause at work is a big issue for many women

I have recently read an interesting article about menopause at work. Here is an excerpt from it:

"We have a "heated global crisis" (pardon the pun) because there are so many baby boomers (women born between 1946-1964) who are "hormonally challenged" and working today.

In fact 6,000 women in the US reach menopause each day. That is roughly, 2 million women per year!!

To better understand and deal with these changes, we must recognize the fact that a great deal of working women prefer to never mention menopause at work. They opt to keep a veil of secrecy surrounding their menopausal experience, even while they may be highly symptomatic during working hours.

In addition, some women go to extreme measures to hide their symptoms. Some women are tremendously embarrassed to openly talk about menopause at work, because of fear of negative comments and/or ridicule associated with symptoms. And, they are also concerned about receiving criticism if they take sick leave due to symptoms.

They also have encountered difficulties about bringing up the "taboo" subject of menopause at work. Communication barriers still exist, causing silence around the subject of menopause."

The U.S. Dept. of Labor statistics indicate that there are over 26.5 million women employed in the U.S. who are between 45 and 64 years of age, of which 15 to 20 million experience menopause symptoms.

It is estimated that 20% of menopausal women experience moderate to severe symptoms. Based on the above figures, between 3 and 5 million American woman are struggling with menopause at work.

A survey of 1,500 working menopausal women, conducted by The Working Mother Research Institute, found that nearly half the women said that managing menopause at work is difficult. They cited hot flashes, changes in memory and concentration and fatigue, due to sleep disturbances, as their most common issues. (173)

Specific findings were the following:

- About one-third cited hot flashes as the most troublesome symptoms in the workplace, and roughly two-thirds said that they occurred daily.
- Changes in memory and concentration and fatigue (attributable to sleep disruption) were also among the most troublesome symptoms.
- Almost half (48%) reported that managing their symptoms took a toll on their work life, with 12% passing up more demanding work or promotions as a result.
- The more 'male' the work environment, the more that women tried to hide their menopausal symptoms while at work; this distinction was almost two-fold.

- Less than one on three women felt comfortable discussing their symptoms with their supervisors and among those who were, again, gender was a strong determining factor.

Recently researchers have examined several aspects of menopause and work in the Women at Work study. (174)

The lead researcher said:

"Businesses plan for younger people to be accommodated through parental leave after the birth of a child, but no provision is made to cope with the problems experienced by women going through symptoms experienced during and after the menopause."

An extensive study conducted in 2010 called Women's Experience of Working through Menopause, found poor concentration, tiredness and poor memory as the top symptoms affecting the performance of menopausal women in the workplace. 78% of the women agreed their job performance had been negatively affected by their menopausal symptoms. 70% of women had not told their managers that they were experiencing menopause. (175)

A major study conducted in 2013 compared menopause symptoms of 17,322 working menopausal women with 17,322 working women who were not menopausal. The results were eye popping.

The menopausal women had significantly higher experiences of depression, anxiety and insomnia, than the working women who were not menopausal. The menopausal women incurred significantly higher medical costs and their productivity was 11% lower, than the non-menopausal group. (176)

So, what do these flashing, fatigued women desire in their work environment? Overwhelmingly, few primary 'want' shines through:

- The ability to adjust the room temperature in their workspace
- A flexible dress code
- Permission to bring and use a fan into the workspace.

By all means, take steps that will help you to manage menopause at work better. But also take steps to relieve those symptoms.

Many women have experienced relief from the symptoms mentioned in the above report, by engaging in self-administered natural progesterone cream. It is an effective, safe and inexpensive treatment for your symptoms.

46

Aging: You See Sagging Skin And Wrinkles ...

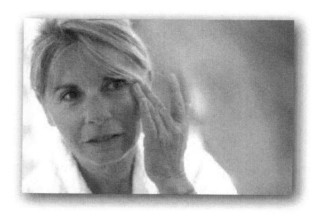

"For the first time in my life, I feel so sick and fragile. Until now, I've never thought of myself as old and I've never given much thought to getting older. And now, I'm suddenly faced with the notion that my body is losing some of its functions and that I've somehow entered a period of physical and mental decline. It is a scary realization."

S. G.

This is what Sharon said ... but the similar thoughts have been expressed by many women during menopause. It is during menopause that many women consider aging for the first time.

There is so much change happening inside your body during menopause. Yet many women are troubled most by what is happening on the outside to their bodies.

Your appearance deteriorates so much during menopause. It makes you look older than you are. Losing your youthful looks can be traumatic in a culture that values appearance over everything.

Aging is like an iceberg. Just a small portion of an iceberg is above the surface and visible. The largest part of an iceberg is below the surface and not visible.

And, so it is with aging. You see the changes in the skin on your face and body. You see sagging boobs. But, you do not see the aging that is occurring internally in the organs of your body. This is where most of your aging is occurring. It has the biggest impact on your health for the rest of your life.

Just as your skin loses its youthfulness as you age, so are the internal organs of your body. Your skin and your internal organs are made of the same ingredient- proteins.

You've probably heard that proteins are important nutrients that help you build muscles. But they are much more than that. Proteins are worker molecules that are necessary for virtually every activity in your body. (177) Collagen is the most abundant protein in your body.

Collagen is also the major component of your hair. Each bulb of hair on your head is surrounded by a sheath of collagen. It helps each strand of hair maintain its thickness and its strength.

Collagen is the main connective tissue that holds you together. It is a vital component of most structures in your body including the following organs and tissues: (178)

Heart, Brain, Gallbladder, Kidneys, Bladder, Digestive tract, Blood vessels, Bones, Muscles, Tendons, Skin, Hair, Nails

It strengthens and protects them. If it weren't for collagen, your body would literally fall apart.

COLLAGEN AND AGING

As you age, the quantity and quality of collagen in your body decreases.

When you were younger, the youthfulness of your skin was attributed to a substance called collagen. Collagen made up 75 percent of your skin. It gave structure to your skin and provided the foundation for the retention of youthful skin. It helped to keep your skin moist and firm. It "held" the skin together. (183)

Collagen is also the major component of your hair. Each bulb of hair on your head is surrounded by a sheath of collagen. It helps each strand of hair maintain its thickness and its strength.

Quantity of collagen:

Your body produces collagen throughout your life, but in decreasing amounts as you age. The decline of collagen production appears to be most rapid in the perimenopause years. (179)

Since the age 30, you've been losing one percent of your collagen a year. The loss of collagen becomes more rapid in the first two years after menopause. 30% percent of your collagen is lost in the first five years after menopause.

Science has long known that estrogen plays a vital role in maintaining the level of collagen in your body. The level of collagen in your body follows the same pattern as the level of estrogen, as you age. Falling estrogen levels = falling collagen levels. (180)

Quality of collagen

There are two processes that are ongoing in your body right now that greatly degrades the quality of collagen in your body and accelerates your aging. They are called glycation and chronic inflammation.

Glycation is a natural process in your body in which glucose attaches to proteins in your body, such as collagen, and form new molecules called advanced glycation end products, or AGEs. These AGEs degrade collagen causing it to harden and lose elasticity in the same way rust weakens and degrades metal.

PROGESTERONE AND AGING

Progesterone does not affect your skin and hair directly, but it affects them indirectly.

Progesterone ensures that the estrogen is received and used by the cells of your skin and hair. Progesterone helps make estrogen receptors more sensitive. An estrogen receptor is a molecule in a cell that makes the cell sensitive to receiving estrogen.

Without sensitive estrogen receptors, your skin and hair cells would not receive estrogen ... even if you had very high levels of it in your body.

Low levels of progesterone during menopause decreases the sensitivity of your skin and hair estrogen receptors, thereby decreasing the level of estrogen in those cells.

TESTOSTERONE AND AGING

Many women are surprised to learn that the female body produces testosterone. They think of it as a male hormone. Your body produces decreasing amounts of it during perimenopause.

However, the level of testosterone in your body during menopause does not fall as much as the level of estrogen. (116)

The higher ratio of testosterone to estrogen is the cause of hair loss. There is a form of testosterone that degrades your hair cells. It is kept in check prior to perimenopause by higher estrogen levels.

The higher ratio of testosterone to estrogen is the cause of acne during menopause. Testosterone is involved in the production of oil by your skin. The higher ratio of testosterone to estrogen causes increased oiliness associated with acne.

THYROID HORMONE AND AGING

26% of menopausal women have an underactive thyroid condition, known as hypothyroidism. It is a condition in which there is insufficient thyroid hormone levels to efficiently manage the metabolism. The metabolism slows. (56)

A slowed metabolism reduces sweating. Skin without enough moisture can quickly become dry and flaky. It leads to itchy skin and other skin complaints. It leads to wrinkles and sagging skin.

Hypothyroidism also causes hair loss. Thyroid hormone is involved in the hair growth cycle. Insufficient thyroid suppresses hair growth and encourages hair to fall out.

CORTISOL AND AGING

Cortisol is the stress hormone. Your body increases production of it during times of stress. Its levels are higher during menopause than prior to it, because the physical, mental and emotional symptoms experienced during menopause result in higher levels of stress for most women.

High levels of cortisol triggers inflammation which breaks down collagen...Resulting in thin skin, fine lines, wrinkles, sagging skin and dryness. It also weakens your hair follicles. (184)

47

You Don't Have to Look Older Than You Are During Menopause

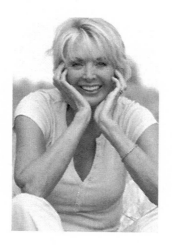

"Suppose that I told you there was a pill that would keep your heart strong, your mind sharp, and your body youthful well into your seventies, eighties, nineties, and even beyond? Suppose that I told you there was a pill that could extend your life and improve your sex life? Suppose I told you there was a pill that could prevent cancer? How about a pill that could keep your skin supple and wrinkle-free? I'm talking about

antioxidants, a family of vitamins, minerals, and other nutrients that I have been studying for the better part of my seventy years."

Dr. Lester Packer

It seems that people have been searching for the fountain of youth forever. Today millions of women use anti-aging products and services in search of a more youthful appearance.

The total market for anti-aging products and services was valued at $249 billion in 2012. Just search Google for anti-aging products and it will reveal 10 million sites about anti-aging products.

Could it be that the answer to anti-aging lies in nature's own substances called antioxidants?

Antioxidants are an antidote for a destructive process that has been ongoing in your body since your birth. Chances are that you are not very familiar with the destructive process.

OXIDATIVE STRESS - AN ONGOING DESTRUCTIVE PROCESS IN YOUR BODY

There is an ongoing destructive process occurring in your body, since birth, called oxidative stress. (185) It has been occurring throughout your life. It is the cause of aging. Many researchers believe that it is a factor behind almost every known disease.

Oxidative stress is exacerbated during perimenopause and post menopause. It is exacerbated by the changes that occur in the ratios of the hormones in your body as a result of menopause. A by-product of this process is something called free radicals.

A free radical is a single electron in an atom of a cell in the body that is looking for a mate. Unlike a stable cell in which every atom is ringed by pairs of electrons, free radicals are cells carrying one or more atoms that have an un-mated electron that desperately wants to pair up with another electron.

The Free radicals "steal" (grab or snatch) an electron from a neighboring cell. (186) This damages the neighboring cell. By snaring an electron from a neighboring cell, it then makes that cell into a free radical. This sets off a chain reaction that wreaks havoc on cells. This chain reaction is called oxidative stress, the cause of aging.

EFFECTS OF OXIDATIVE STRESS ON YOUR BODY

It is important to note that damage from oxidative stress accumulates with age, just like the discoloration you see when an apple slice is left out in the air.

Oxidative stress is associated with the symptoms and infirmities of aging. One of its most visible symptoms is dryness in the skin, causing lines and wrinkles on the face and body.

There are a host of other symptoms of oxidative stress that contribute to aging and age related ailments, and life threatening diseases.

ANTIOXIDANTS – NATURE'S ANTI-AGING SUBSTANCE

Antioxidants are substances made by our bodies, and nutrients found in food, that stop the spread of free radicals. In so doing, they are very effective anti-aging agents. (187)

When an antioxidant encounters a free radical it freely gives up an electron of its own, which satisfies the free radical and stops the out of control damage. This makes the antioxidant a free radical because it's now an electron short. However, the chain reaction is stopped because the newly created free radical made from the antioxidant is very weak and unlikely to do further harm.

Apart from making you look younger, or at least your actual age, they are an antidote for the infirmities associated with aging – including life threatening diseases.

There is considerable evidence from studies that indicates that antioxidants can slow or prevent the development of cancer. (188)

According to a recent study in The American Journal of Medicine, antioxidants can greatly reduce the risk of heart attack in women. (189)

It is important to note that these health benefits come from the natural antioxidants found in food. Studies have found that antioxidants taken as supplements do not reduce the risk of cancer or heart attack.

THE ANTI-AGING ANTIOXIDANTS
Some antioxidants are made by your body. These include Coenzyme Q10 (CoQ 10), Alpha-Lipoic Acid, Glutathione and Melatonin.

Other antioxidants come from the intake of food. They are abundant in fresh fruits and vegetables, as well as in other natural *un-processed* foods including nuts, grains and some meats, poultry and fish. The list below describes food sources of common antioxidants

1. Beta-carotene – found in many foods that are orange in color, including sweet potatoes, carrots, cantaloupe, squash, apricots, pumpkin, and mangos. Some green leafy vegetables including collard greens, spinach, and kale are also rich in beta-carotene.
2. Lutein – is abundant in green, leafy vegetables such as collard greens, spinach, and kale.
3. Lycopene – found in tomatoes, watermelon, guava, papaya, apricots, pink grapefruit, blood oranges, and other foods.
4. Selenium – it is a mineral, not an antioxidant nutrient. However, it is a component of antioxidant enzymes. Found in rice and wheat products, meat and Brazil nuts.
5. Vitamin A – Foods rich in vitamin A include liver, sweet potatoes, carrots, milk, egg yolks and mozzarella cheese.
6. Vitamin C – found in high abundance in many fruits and vegetables and is also found in cereals, beef, poultry and fish.
7. Vitamin E – found in almonds, in many oils including wheat germ, safflower, corn and soybean oils, and also found in mangos, nuts, and broccoli.

48

Aging: Vanity Is The Least Of Your Concerns ....
How To Reduce The REAL Threat

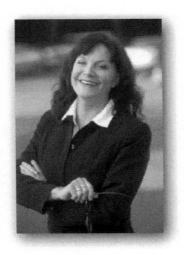

"And the beauty of a woman, with passing years only grows!"

AUDREY HEPBURN

Aging is a natural part of life. It can't be reversed, but it can be slowed down.

In midlife there are days when looking in the mirror feels like life has suddenly played a very cruel trick. The picture in your mind's eye does not always match the image staring back at you.

It's no secret that we live in a youth-obsessed culture. We are bombarded daily with images via movies, television, magazines, billboards, and the internet. It's all about the look and the image.

It is not surprising that the total global market for anti-aging products and services was valued at $261.9 billion in 2013.

A recent survey of 2,000 women found that (190):

- 56 percent of women are worried about the physical signs of aging.
- 42 percent of women admitted they'd undergo plastic surgery or resort to anti-aging injections to keep signs of aging at bay.
- 41% of women wish they looked younger.
- Women think that wrinkles are the most revealing sign of a woman's age.

This preoccupation with our appearance camouflages and obfuscates the REAL threat of aging, life threatening diseases that are caused by two ongoing processes in the body and are associated with aging. The two processes are called glycation and chronic inflammation.

The impact of these processes and the risk of life threatening diseases can be reduced.

Before providing you with an overview of these processes, it is first necessary that you have some information about a major component of your body- Collagen.

COLLAGEN IS THE MOST ABUNDANT PROTEIN IN YOUR BODY
Collagen is the main connective tissue that holds you together. (178) It is a vital component of most structures in your body including your heart, brain, gallbladder, kidneys, bladder, digestive tract, blood vessels, bones, muscles, tendons, skin, hair, nails.

As you age, the quality of the collagen in your body is degraded by glycation and chronic inflammation.

WHAT IS GLYCATION?

Glycation is a natural process in your body in which glucose attaches to proteins in your body, such as collagen, and form new molecules called advanced glycation end products, or AGEs. These AGEs degrade collagen causing it to harden and lose elasticity in the same way rust weakens and degrades metal. (181)

The sequence of events leading to formation of AGEs goes like this: Ingest foods that increase blood glucose.

The greater availability of glucose to the body's tissues permits the glucose molecule to react with any protein, creating a combined glucose-protein molecule.

Once AGEs form, they are irreversible and cannot be undone. AGE is resistant to any of the body's digestive or cleansing processes.

AGEs cause aging. They weaken every system in your body by degrading the collagen in those systems.

CHRONIC INFLAMMATION AND AGING

It all starts with the immune system, your body's first line of defense against any kind of harm. When you're injured or ill, your body dispatches white blood cells to root out the harmful stimuli and jump-start the healing process. When the threat has been dealt with, the inflammation process ends.

As discussed previously, Chronic "hidden" inflammation occurs throughout your body when something kick-starts the immune system and disengages the shut-off button. The white blood cells are mobilized and they end up just hanging around, often for a long, long time. The white blood cells attack (inflame) healthy tissue (collagen), causing it to degrade.

Chronic inflammation has many triggers. Glycation is one of them.

Chronic inflammation is hidden. You won't feel pain or feel sick initially, but a fire is quietly smoldering within you, upsetting the delicate balance among all of the major systems of your body ... endocrine, central nervous, digestive, and cardiovascular/respiratory.

DISEASES CAUSED BY GLYCATION AND CHRONIC INFLAMMATION

Glycation and chronic inflammation are destructive to your health and well-being. It contributes to disease and age-related deterioration such as:

- cancer
- heart disease
- stroke
- Alzheimer's Disease
- diabetes
- arthritis
- osteoporosis
- all autoimmune diseases

How to reduce the effects of glycation and chronic inflammation on your body, and slow down aging:

- Eliminate fast foods and processed foods from your diet. There is added sugar in these foods to enhance their flavor. Also, food manufacturers have added AGEs to these foods, especially in the last 50 years, as flavor enhancers and colorants to improve flavor AND appearance.

A diet in which fast food and processed food is present will keep your glucose (blood sugar) level high, which fosters glycation and chronic inflammation.

Base your diet around fresh and non-process food to reduce glycation and chronic inflammation. Increase your intake of unprocessed meat, fish, milk, eggs, legumes, fruits, grains and vegetables.

- Reduce the amount of food that you cook using dry heat methods – including barbecuing, grilling, frying, sautéing, broiling, searing and toasting.

A study has found that when food is cooked using high levels of dry heat, the AGE content of the food skyrockets. (191)

Moist cooking methods such as boiling, steaming, poaching, stewing or simmering does not create AGEs.

- Get your vitamin D tested. Many people today are deficient in vitamin D. Vitamin D is essential to the healthy functioning of all systems of your body. Deficiency of vitamin D fosters glycation and chronic inflammation.

49

Women Are Deficient In Progesterone From The Age Of 35

PROGESTERONE IS A VERY SPECIAL HORMONE

Doctors know that it becomes increasingly difficult for a woman to become pregnant after the age of 35. One of the reasons may be due to falling progesterone levels from the age of 35. (192)

Progesterone is "the pregnancy hormone," it is essential before and during pregnancy. All women who wish to become pregnant need progesterone to help the uterus prepare for and maintain a fertilized egg.

After ovulation occurs, the ovaries start to produce progesterone needed by the uterus. It causes the uterine lining or endometrium to thicken. This helps prepare a supportive environment in the uterus for a fertilized egg.

The most common cause of age-related decline in fertility is less frequent ovulation. (193) As women age, they begin to have occasional cycles where an egg is never released. This is caused by decreasing quality and quantity of a woman's eggs in her 30s and 40s.

Anovulation (a menstrual cycle during which the ovaries do not release an egg) is the cause of irregular periods during perimenopause. It occurs increasingly as a woman progresses through perimenopause toward post menopause. It is the cause of continuously falling progesterone levels during perimenopause.

Falling levels of progesterone has an adverse effect on the healthy functioning of your body. It also directly causes some of the menopause symptoms that you are experiencing. It also, together with fluctuating estrogen levels, causes all the rest of the menopause symptoms not caused by falling progesterone levels.

HOW PROGESTERONE KEEPS YOUR BODY HEALTHY?

Progesterone is a very special hormone (194). Its many functions in the body include:

- Keeping your nervous system functioning as it should. It helps to develop the protective sheath around every nerve in your body. It also repairs the sheath when it is damaged by illness or injury.
- Increasing metabolism and promoting weight loss.
- Helping your brain to function as it should. It improves verbal memory and overall cognitive function.
- Alleviating depression and reducing anxiety.
- Balancing blood sugar levels.
- Normalizing blood clotting.
- Stimulating the production of new bone. It helps to prevent osteo-arthritis and osteoporosis.
- Protecting the heart in many ways, including its ability to reduce high blood pressure.
- Promoting normal sleep patterns. It is called the "soporific hormone".
- Keeping your libido healthy. Falling progesterone levels cause loss of libido.
- Keeping your hair healthy. Falling levels of progesterone is the cause of menopause hair loss. Hair loss is reversed by progesterone therapy, which increases the level of progesterone in your body.
- Helping to keep your skin healthy. Low progesterone levels causes acne and other skin complaints.

Menopause symptoms directly attributed to progesterone deficiency (195):

- Anxiety
- Irritability
- Hypersensitivity
- Nervousness
- Restless sleep
- Headaches/migraines before menstruation
- Weight gain
- Breast tenderness
- Decreased libido
- Heavy periods

All of the other menopause symptoms are caused by a combination of the changing levels of both progesterone and estrogen during perimenopause.

Prior to perimenopause, all of the hormones in your body work in harmony by co-existing with one another in a certain ratio. They are said to be balanced. This keeps your body healthy and functioning.

HOW TO RESTORE PROGESTERONE TO A HEALTHY LEVEL AND MAINTAIN IT?

1. Traditional HRT
2. Bio-identical hormone therapy (BHRT). However, it is an expensive treatment and most health insurance policies do not cover it.
3. Self-administered bioidentical progesterone cream. It raises the level of progesterone in your body, while bringing estrogen into greater balance with it. It is safe, effective and inexpensive treatment.

A Mayo Clinic study (196) that examined the effectiveness of bio-identical progesterone therapy found that it brought about a:

- 30% reduction in sleep problems
- 50% reduction in anxiety
- 60% reduction in depression
- 25% reduction in menstrual bleeding
- 40% reduction in cognitive difficulties
- 30% improvement in sexual function

CHOOSE YOUR PROGESTERONE CAREFULLY

There are many forms of progesterone. They are not all equal in terms of effectiveness and safety:

1. Beware of Progestin. They are a synthetic version of progesterone used by pharma companies in their HRT products. They do not function the same way in your body as progesterone. They were added to estrogen in hrt products to prevent endometrial cancer, which was found to be prevalent in women who used estrogen HRT.

2. Beware of creams that do not say USP progesterone cream on the label.

   The term 'USP' refers to the grade or purity of the product and is the shortened form of the term 'United States Pharmacopeia'. There are three different grades of raw materials used in products – 'USP pharmaceutical grade', 'food grade' for human consumption and 'feed grade' that is for animal consumption.

   USP natural progesterone refers to the progesterone substance that is exactly the same hormone that is made by the human body.

3. Beware of wild yam creams. They are passed off as progesterone cream. Here is what WebMD says about wild yam creams:

"Although wild yam cream is marketed as a source of natural progesterone, it does not contain progesterone, and the body cannot convert it into progesterone."

A study published in the American Journal of Obstetrics and Gynecology found that the creams made from wild yams are not metabolized to progesterone by women. (197)

4. Beware of progesterone creams that contain too little progesterone. The cream needs to have an adequate amount of progesterone in it.

Harvard-trained physician Dr. John R. Lee, the pioneer researcher of progesterone therapy, wrote that natural progesterone cream should contain 2%-3% USP natural progesterone per ounce of cream.

50

How to Nurture A Positive Attitude Toward Menopause

"Keep your face always toward the sunshine - and shadows will fall behind you."

WALT WHITMAN

Menopause has been easier for me since I stopped being angry about it It is entirely possible that your attitude to menopause would be different, if you were living in another country.

We tend to take it for granted that all women, everywhere in the world, experience menopause in a way that is similar to the way in which we experience it.

This is probably because we're so used to hearing the representation of menopause, by the medical community, as a disease with symptoms that require a doctor's treatment. If it is a disease, women everywhere would experience it in a similar way.

However menopause is not a disease and in various cultures, that are different from our own, it is experienced very differently from the way in which you experience it.

In the US, the symptom that troubles women the most is hot flashes. Approximately 75% of American women experience them.

By contrast, it couldn't be more different in Asia. Hot flashes have been reported by only about 10 percent of women in China, 17 percent of women in Singapore, and 25 percent of women in Japan.

In 2006 the results of an international survey of menopausal women, to find the symptom that troubled them the most, was reported.

Women from Indonesia, Japan, Korea, Lebanon, Malaysia, Mexico, Philippines, Singapore, Taiwan and Thailand as well as US, UK, Australia, Canada, Finland and Hong Kong were polled.

When the results were examined collectively, the symptom that troubled women the most was not hot flashes, but headaches. After headaches came joint problems, irritability, lack of energy and nervous tension.

CULTURAL ATTITUDES TO MENOPAUSE

Is it possible that the attitude to menopause in different countries and cultures, has a bearing on how women in those cultures experience menopause?

In America, and in western societies, women tend to be valued for their physical and sexual attractiveness, reproductive capacity and youthfulness.

Their role, which is constantly being re-enforced by Hollywood, television, and the advertising industry, is to remain beautiful, attractive and supportive of their family.

These are valuable traits, but what happens to women when her breasts sag, her skin wrinkles and her children leave home to live their own lives?

Aging is often viewed negatively, and with distaste, among women and society at large. Many women are terrified of it. Menopause is viewed as a sign of aging.

In America, menopause is largely viewed negatively as the end of menstruation and with it the beginning of gradual decline into an "all downhill from here" state of mind. Older people are not valued. They are more likely to be shunted to a scrap heap by society at large.

In many other cultures, menopause is viewed positively, as a transition to new phase in life, where the women are valued for her wisdom. She becomes a valued elder of the family and society.

In Japan the word for menopause is konenki. Literally translated, KO means "renewal and regeneration," NEN means "year" or "years," and Ki means "season" or "energy."

In these cultures, women experience less menopausal symptoms which suggest women's attitudes to menopause can act as self-fulfilling prophecies.

Could it be that the prevailing attitude in America to menopause is a self-fulfilling prophesy, as well?

Could it be that many American women suffer the symptoms they experience, because of their attitude to menopause and aging?

An MD at the highly respected Cleveland Clinic's Women's Health Institute says (198):

"Embracing this time in your life rather than dreading it can make such a big difference in how you experience menopause. Anthropological studies of various cultures suggest that how you go through this life stage is largely dependent on your attitude."

HERE IS WHAT YOU CAN DO TO NURTURE A POSITIVE ATTITUDE TO MENOPAUSE:

- Become informed about the menopause attitudes and experiences of women from all over the world.
- Use an anti-stress technique, such as yoga, meditation etc., regularly.
- Proactively seek remedies, which are consistent with your values that will relieve the symptoms you are experiencing.
- Foster/strengthen relationships with women who have a positive attitude to menopause. Those relationships can be with friends already in your life or with "online friends".
- Embrace change. Let go of the past. Create your future and pursue it with enthusiasm.
- Benefit from a daily exercise.
- Your attitude to menopause can lift you up or it can bring you down. The choice is yours!

Maybe a few more...
Shades of Menopause

Hormonal Replacement
Therapy- HRT

Is Hormone Replacement A Good Idea?
Who Says What...?

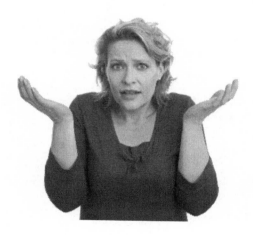

The information about HRT is so confusing

A debate has raged for 70 years as to whether or not menopausal women should replace their sex hormones. There is so much conflicting data around this debate, that it confuses most women.

Prior to 2002, millions of women used hormone replacement because it promised age-reversal and it was effective at relieving hot flashes, night sweats and the vaginal atrophy that caused vaginal dryness and pain during sexual intercourse.

Then in 2002, the findings of the landmark WHI study were released. It showed that the most common form of hormone replacement therapy – estrogen and synthetic progestin – increased a woman's risk of breast cancer, heart attack and stroke.

As a result, the use of all forms of hormone replacement therapy decreased to a small fraction of what it had been.

In the ensuing years since the release of the WHI findings, pharma and leading medical bodies have acknowledged the increased health risks associated with taking estrogen plus progestin.

In so doing, they have also argued that the increased health risks are relatively small and that the benefits to women, who experience severe menopause symptoms, outweigh the risks.

It may appear to women who experience severe menopause symptoms, that the question that they need to answer is … which is more important to them

Quality of life now vs. long term future health
This is so unfair. Clearly women would like to have both. Perhaps there is way to achieve both.

The term hormone replacement, or HRT, is used to describe two distinctly different forms of therapies

1. Traditional hormone replacement prescribed by most medical practitioners.
2. Bioidentical hormone replacement therapy.

It muddies the water to refer to both as hormone replacement therapy. While both do replace hormones, they are as different as apples and oranges. For the sake of clarity, I will refer to traditional hormone replacement therapy as HRT and bioidentical hormone therapy as BHRT.

HRT covers estrogen (estradiol and estrone) therapy and estrogen plus progestin therapy. Progestin is a drug that tries to mimic natural progesterone. BHRT covers estrogen therapy (estriol) and natural progesterone therapy.

PROS AND CONS OF HRT

Proponents of HRT (199) say that it helps to relieve menopause symptoms and reduces the risk of osteoporosis. They say that it causes a slight increased risk of breast cancer, heart attack and stroke.

Opponents of HRT (199) say that synthetic estrogen (estradiol and estrone) reduces hot flashes, night sweats, vaginal dryness and the risk of osteoporosis and heart disease, while increasing the risks of breast and uterine cancer, stroke, liver and gall bladder disease and fibroids. The say that progestin decreases the risk of uterine cancer...but increases the risk of breast cancer.

LEF – The Life Extension Foundation – says that a combined analysis from 27 published studies of HRT reveals a 28% reduction in mortality in menopausal women under age 60 who replace their sex hormones. The studies also show profound quality of life improvements in hormone-replenished women. (200)

LEF is one of the largest organizations dedicated to investigating every method of extending the healthy human life span. It is a nonprofit, tax-exempt organization.

LEF recommends BHRT in preference to HRT. It says that the health risks associated with HRT comes from two drugs:

"In their panic to "do no harm," conventional doctors minimized all sex hormone prescribing. Yet the two drugs specifically linked to increase cancer and vascular risks in the Women's Health Initiative trial data were PremPro® and Premarin®.

Premarin® is a horse urine-derived drug that contains some estrogens that are unnatural to the human body. It is avoided by enlightened women and some doctors today, but is still the most frequently prescribed oral estrogen drug.

PremPro® is a combination of Premarin® and a synthetic progestin. This progestin, called medroxyprogesterone, is not the same compound as the natural progesterone it was supposed to function as.

A review of the published literature reveals that progestin is a major culprit behind the higher rates of vascular disease and cancer that caused doctors to abandon all female hormone drugs beginning in 2002-2004."

Pros and cons of BHRT cite an article by Dr. Follingstad in the Journal of the American Medical Association in which he says that estriol is as effective as estradiol and estrone in relieving menopause symptoms and does not bear their carcinogenic effects.

With respect to bioidentical progesterone vs progestin, proponents cite a Mayo Clinic study of 176 menopausal women who took bioidentical progesterone, after having previously taken HRT (estradiol and estrone plus progestin). (196) The beneficial effects of bioidentical progesterone compared to progestin included a

- 30% reduction in sleep problems
- 50% reduction in anxiety
- 60% reduction in depression
- 25% reduction in menstrual bleeding
- 40% reduction in cognitive difficulties
- 30% improvement in sexual function

Proponents of BHRT also cite studies that found that bioidentical progesterone reduces the risks of breast cancer, heart attack and stroke, while HRT with progestin increases these risks.

Opponents of BHRT state that there have not been any clinical trials to establish the safety record of BHRT, only observational studies.

Medical science favors clinical trials over observational studies. Proponents of BHRT counter this argument by saying that all clinical trials are funded by pharma, and pharma are not about to fund BHRT trials.

They say that BHRT is the competition to pharma HRT products. They also state that pharma cannot patent **natural** BHRT" products.... because they can't make money from them.

HRT vs. Going Natural – Which Way Is Better?

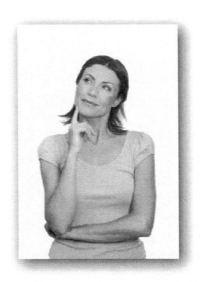

Which way is better for me?

This question can generate an emotional, and often heated, response from advocates on both sides. HRT is controversial. Some say that it has saved their lives. Others say it can kill.

Some advocates of the natural route suggest that it is nobler to go natural. They imply that it is a matter of personal strength and that those who take HRT are weaker than those you go natural. Some advocates of HRT are incensed by attitudes like this.

WHAT HAS BROUGHT ABOUT THIS DIVIDE?

HRT (synthetic hormone products manufactured by pharmaceutical companies) is effective at relieving many of the menopause symptoms. 13 million women in America were taking it to relieve their menopause symptoms, until the 2002 findings of the WHI study, which examined health risks associated with taking HRT, were announced. It was the favored treatment for menopause symptoms.

The WHI study found that the increase in the relative risk for breast cancer was 26%, for heart attack 29%, for stroke 41%, and for blood clots 100%. Since that time less than 20% of menopausal women take HRT. (201)

Since the release of these findings, sales of HRT products by pharma companies have plummeted. Pharma companies have resorted to using unscrupulous marketing techniques in an attempt to boost sales. (202)

These marketing techniques were brought to light during court cases against pharma companies, brought by women who have experienced serious health problems as a result of taking HRT.

The media revelation of the use of these unscrupulous marketing techniques by pharma, plus the revelation in the media that most OB-GYNs do not receive training about menopause and do not understand it, causes many women to be suspicious when doctors recommend HRT for their menopause symptoms. (203)

Since 2002, women, who are concerned about the health risks of taking HRT, have been looking for "natural" treatments for menopause symptoms that are free of these health risks. "Natural" treatments are classified as CAM (complementary and alternative medicine) and holistic medicine.

CAM is an acronym for complementary and alternative medicine. Complementary medicine is used together with conventional medicine, and alternative medicine is used in place of conventional medicine. (204)

Holistic medicine is also referred to as integrative medicine. (205) Holistic medicine physicians combine conventional and CAM treatments. Many holistic physicians also prescribe BHRT to treat menopause symptoms.

Advocates of BHRT say that bioidentical hormones are natural and that they exactly duplicate the hormones that are produced by your body. They say that it without the health risks associated with taking synthetic HRT, but this has not been verified by studies.

However proponents of HRT present the argument that their synthetic HRT products are natural, as well. Some advocates of the natural approach to menopause consider BHRT as natural; others consider it to be part of HRT. (206)

How to Evaluate the Risks of Taking HRT

"Citing the WHI for Hormone Replacement Therapy standards equates with attending the Flat Earth Society Conference and listening to people tries to prove the earth is flat."

MARIE HOAG MBA

HRT is such an emotive topic. Just the mention of it in the title of this post, will result in some women not reading this post.

I understand this kind of response. Some women view it as a life saver; others view it as a killer.

Almost every menopausal woman is aware that there is health risks associated with taking hormone replacement therapy. Studies have found that taking it, increases the risk of breast cancer, heart disease and stroke.

Most women elect not to take it, because of those health risks.

However, 7% of menopausal women report that their symptoms have a very negative effect on their lives. It is estimated that there are 50 million menopausal women in America today. 7% of them = 3.5 million women. (207)

For many of these women, their symptoms can be so debilitating that they are unable to function in life adequately.

Their symptoms can have a devastating effect on their roles as a mother, wife, care for elderly parents, and earner of income for the family. Their symptoms, if untreated, can also lead to conditions that can be damaging to their health and well-being, i.e. depression.

For these women, there are risks in not treating their severe symptoms.

Conventional HRT and bioidentical HRT are effective at relieving menopause symptoms.

You will read and hear many competing claims and statistics about hormone replacement therapy. Some doctors say that the benefits outweigh the risks; others say the reverse. Authority sites will tell you to discuss it with your doctor, but in so doing, the answer that you get will be an opinion....that may not even be based on medical fact, but rather the promotional marketing of HRT by a pharma.

WHAT SHOULD YOU DO?

The best and safest thing for you to do is to research the facts yourself. You need to learn how to interpret the research that has been conducted into hormone replacement therapy.

How to evaluate HRT, if you are experiencing debilitating symptoms

To view this matter objectively, you have to look closely at statistics, rather than listen to authors of articles that say "HRT increases the risk of...." or "HRT decreases the risk of...."

We get most of the information about hormone replacement therapy from the media, who report the findings of medical studies.

The headlines and stories will often talk about a "25% increase in risk" of a "25% decrease in risk" etc. But what does this actually mean?

"Risk" in the health and medical fields have special meanings. Knowing the basic types of risk can help you understand your risks in taking HRT.

As you probably know, the big study that first identified the health risks associated with HRT was the 2002 Women's' Health Initiative (WHI). It followed 16,000 women for approximately 5 years. Some of the women took HRT and some did not.

Researchers reported that HRT increased the risk of breast cancer by 26 per cent. That sounds terrifyingly high. But on further inspection this statistic is not quite what it appears to be.

There are different ways of presenting a health risk. For example, if the risk of having a stroke is 2 in 100, and a medication increases it to 3 in 100, then it could be said that the treatment has increased the risk of a stroke by 1 per cent. This method of presenting data is called the absolute risk. (208)

However, it could equally be said that it has increased the risk of a stroke by 50 per cent. While this sounds far more alarming, it is the same data, just presented in a different way. This is called relative risk. (209)

It compares the risk between 2 groups. The WHI study reported findings based on relative risk. It compared the findings of women who took hormone replacement therapy and women who did not.

The relative risk doesn't help you assess the actual risk of a woman on HRT developing breast cancer – because it doesn't tell you how many women would develop breast cancers, which were not on HRT.

In the case of breast cancer and hormone replacement therapy, while the relative risk is 26 per cent, the absolute risk is 0.4 per cent. This means that, according to the WHI study, there are four extra cases of breast cancer per 1,000 women taking it over a five-year period. While this is still significant, it's a clear example of how the same data can be expressed in different ways.

The way that risk information is presented can influence your decision to take HRT or not. (210)

Estrogen – The Angel of Death

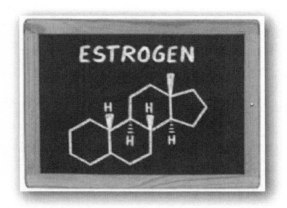

"If I hear of one more articles sourcing the WHI as the standard by which hormone replacement therapy advice should be generated, I think I'm going to puke."

MARIE HOAG MBA

Estrogen can run amuck without progesterone!
In the earlier years of your life, estrogen had a positive impact on your life. It gives much to a woman's life in her earlier years.

However, during the menopause years, when estrogen levels are lower and the ratio between it and progesterone have been altered, estrogen can run amuck. Progesterone counter balances negative effects of estrogen.

With insufficient progesterone to keep it in check, it can cause blood clots, heart disease, strokes and it can create and aid the generation and growth of cancerous cells. For this reason it has been called the angel of death.

Dr Ercole Cavalieri, a scientist who spent 30 years studying the effects of estrogen, has dubbed it the angel of life and the angel of death. He dubbed it such because of the tremendous range of effects – from beneficial to harmful – of estrogen.

ANGEL OF DEATH EFFECTS OF ESTROGEN

The angel of death effects are not a concern, for the most part, until a woman reaches the menopause years.

It becomes a concern then, because that part of a woman's life is associated with symptoms that are attributed to lower levels of estrogen in her body.

Many women, particularly those who experience moderate to severe symptoms, turn to HRT for relief. It is effective at bringing symptom relief.

The most significant component of most types of HRT is estrogen. Two of the most commonly used types of HRT are estrogen only and estrogen + progestin (a synthetic drug that supposedly does what progesterone does). Both of these types of HRT carry angel of death effects.

The angel of death effects is a concern for a woman who has her uterus intact. Studies have found that women who have had a hysterectomy face virtually no HRT health risks.

In fact one large government study found that women who had hysterectomy and who used hormones had a lower risk of breast cancer than women who did not take hormones of any kind. (211)

The following health risks are associated with taking synthetic estrogen only (estrogen replacement therapy), if your uterus is still intact:

- Taking estrogen alone causes the lining of the uterus to grow. The risk for endometrial cancer is six to eight times higher in women who take estrogen, compared with those who do not. One study showed that about 1 in 9 women treated with estrogen only for 3 years, developed a type of pre-cancerous change in the lining of their uterus. (212)

- Postmenopausal women who take estrogen only HRT have 2 – 4 times greater risk of developing a blood clot than women who do not take HRT. However the absolute risk of a blood clot is relatively small ... less than 1%. (213)
- Estrogen only replacement therapy slightly increases the risk of stroke. (214)

Because of the increased risk of endometrial cancer when taking estrogen only HRT, a type of HRT was developed that has eliminated the risk of endometrial cancer....estrogen + progestin (synthetic progesterone).

It is often called combined HRT. However, by adding progestin women have been experiencing other risks to their health. The following health risks are associated with taking estrogen + progestin:

- Current or recent past users of hormonal replacement therapy (HRT) have a higher risk of being diagnosed with breast cancer. Combination HRT increases breast cancer risk by about 75%, even when used for only a short time. (215) Combination HRT also increases the likelihood that the cancer may be found at a more advanced stage, as well as increasing the risk that a woman diagnosed with breast cancer will die from the disease.

The lead researcher of a 2010 study that examined health risks associated with combined HRT said:

"If combined hormone therapy were a new drug, it's hard to see how you could get it approved." Dr. Rowan T. Chlebowski

- There is no question that HRT significantly increases the risk of forming blood clots in arteries and veins in post-menopausal women.

The WHI study showed a 41% increase in strokes among the women taking estrogen/progestin. For every 10,000 women taking HRT, 29 will have a stroke, compared with 21 in 10,000 women not taking HRT. (212)

- The increased risk of forming blood clots in arteries and veins also increases the risk of heart attack

There have been no clinical trials to examine health risks associated with bioidentical hormone replacement therapy (BHRT).

However a large observational study, involving 100,000 women who were followed for 10 years, found that women using synthetic HRT had an increased risk of breast cancer, while bioidentical hormone users had the same breast cancer risk as women who did not take hormones at all. (216)

A comprehensive analysis of 200 studies showed that taking bioidentical hormones carries a reduced risk of stroke and heart attack. (217)

Not All HRT Increases Your Health Risks ...
Just Some

Is there a proven SAFE way to relieve menopause symptoms?
Many women are too frightened to take HRT, despite experiencing debilitating menopause symptoms that significantly reduces their quality of life. They are frightened because of the negativity associated with the term "HRT". They endure their symptoms.

HRT is an umbrella term for several different kinds of hormone replacement therapy. Some forms of HRT have been proven to increase the risks of heart disease, stroke and cancer. Other forms of HRT have shown no signs of increasing health risks at all.

Just suppose that forms of natural HRT exist, and that they are associated with no future health risks. Would you be prepared to learn about them and possibly use them to relieve your symptoms?

There are two broad types of HRT:

1. Traditional HRT – this type of HRT is a synthetic product. The basis of this product is pregnant mares' urine. The most well-known brand is Premarin (Pre for pregnant – Mar for mares – in for urine). Traditional HRT is what is prescribed by most doctors. Use of it is encouraged by the traditional medical community.

Traditional HRT is effective for the relief of hot flashes, night sweats and vaginal discomfort. It is prescribed mainly to relieve those symptoms. There is no evidence that it effectively relieves other menopause symptoms.

The hormones in traditional HRT products are not identical to the hormones in your body. Your body does not react to them in the same way that it reacts to the natural hormones made by your body.

2. Bioidentical HRT – this type of HRT utilizes hormones that are identical to the hormones made by your body. Your body reacts to bioidentical hormones in the same way that it reacts to the hormones made by your body.

Bioidentical HRT effectively relieves hot flashes, night sweats, heavy menstrual bleeding, mood swings, anxiety, menopause headaches, disturbed sleep, breast tenderness, cognitive difficulties (memory loss, fuzzy thinking, and difficulties concentrating) and other symptoms.

HEALTH RISKS ASSOCIATED WITH TAKING TRADITIONAL HRT

Traditional HRT can be taken in two forms: estrogen progestin (progestin is a synthetic drug that supposedly does what progesterone does ….but it doesn't!) and estrogen only.

Estrogen progestin is the form of traditional that is used the most by women. Medical studies have found that it increases the risk of breast cancer, heart attack, stroke and blood clots in women who take it. (218)

Estrogen alone is only safe for women who do not have a uterus. In women who still have a uterus, using estrogen only has been shown to increase the risk of blood clots, stroke and endometrial cancer. (219)

According to the National Cancer Institute, there can be no doubt that taking traditional HRT, in the form of synthetic estrogen plus progestin or synthetic estrogen only, increases the risks of breast cancer, heart attack and stroke. (220)

Because of the health risks associated with taking traditional HRT, doctors recommend that it be taken for the shortest amount of time in the lowest possible dosage. It is recommended to take it for no longer than 5 years. This in itself poses a problem for users of traditional HRT.

Women, who are most likely to take traditional HRT, suffer with moderate to severe hot flashes and night sweats. Several studies have found that many women with severe to moderate hot flashes experience them for 10 years or longer. One major study found that the average duration is 10 years. (221)

What should a woman do if she experiences moderate to severe hot flashes that can last for around 10 years, but should only take traditional HRT for up to 5 years?

A second issue facing women who take traditional HRT is what happens when she stops taking traditional HRT. A study of 8,400 postmenopausal women found that more than half of the women, who started taking traditional HRT to relieve symptoms of menopause, saw a dramatic resurgence of those symptoms when they discontinued the therapy. (222)

No known health risks associated with taking Bioidentical HRT.

There are two forms of bioidentical HRT:

1. You can get the levels of your hormones tested and then re-balanced by a hormone expert. The hormone expert will prescribe the exact levels of each hormone needed to re-balance them.
2. You can use progesterone therapy – progesterone therapy entails the self-application of bio-identical progesterone cream. This raises your progesterone level while lowering your estrogen level, thereby relieving your symptoms. Perimenopause symptoms are caused by too little progesterone in your body....relative to the amount of estrogen.

Studies have found no evidence that bioidentical HRT causes any health risks. Accordingly, there is no need to restrict the use of it to 5 years, as is the case with traditional HRT. You can take bioidentical HRT for as long as you have menopause symptoms.

There is no need to suffer with severe symptoms. You can relieve them with bioidentical HRT ... without increasing your health risks.

Perimenopause Symptoms...Made Worse by a Devil You Don't Know

Why you are recommending HRT?

Most women think that their perimenopause symptoms are caused by insufficient estrogen in their bodies. This is incorrect.

Contrary to what you may have been led to believe, perimenopause symptoms are caused by too much estrogen in your body and not enough progesterone.

Estrogen levels are actually higher during early perimenopause than they are in pre-premenopausal women. (7)

While estrogen levels rise in early perimenopause, progesterone levels fall. (223) Progesterone levels continue to fall throughout late perimenopause. Estrogen levels fall later in perimenopause, but not as much as progesterone, thus, changes the ratio between these two hormones.

Estrogen becomes dominant. (224)

Estrogen dominance disturbs the balance between all the other hormones in your body. As your hormones collectively control all of the processes in your body, the processes behave erratically. The result is the symptoms that you are experiencing.

Traditional HRT worsens perimenopause symptoms.

Most doctors recommend and prescribe traditional HRT to relieve perimenopause symptoms. The most significant component of traditional

HRT is estrogen. The two most commonly prescribed types of traditional HRT are estrogen only and estrogen + progestin. If your treat your perimenopause symptoms with traditional HRT, you will increase the level of estrogen in your body.

As your body already has too much estrogen, relative to progesterone, treating perimenopause symptoms with traditional HRT will worsen your symptoms.

So, why do doctors recommend traditional HRT for perimenopause symptoms?

Most doctors do not understand menopause. This has been established by research conducted by Johns Hopkins Medical School in 2013. (203)

As a result, the primary source of their information about menopause, and the treatment of its symptoms, comes from pharmaceutical companies.

The pharma industry has been aggressively and unscrupulously marketing HRT as THE solution for menopausal women for the past 50 years. They have invested billions of dollars in research and development of their HRT products and they have made billions of dollars from them.

HOW DOES THE PHARMA INDUSTRY EDUCATE DOCTORS ABOUT MENOPAUSE?

To fully understand the answer to this question, I suggest that you read the following articles:

1. Menopause, as Brought to You by Big Pharma – a New York Times expose about the marketing of menopause by pharma. (225)
2. Promotional Tone in Reviews of Menopausal Hormone Therapy after the Women's Health Initiative: An Analysis of Published Articles – a medical study, led by a prominent OB-GYN that is easy for the lay person to understand. (226)

Here is a synopsis of how the pharma companies have "educated" doctors about menopause:

- Ghostwriting – ghostwriting involves writing an article in the name of an "authority", who is paid for lending his/her name to the article. Pharma companies employed specialist firms to write articles that promoted the benefits of their products, without mentioning the risks and side effects.

  They paid prominent doctors and medical professors to allow the articles to be published in their names. These articles (227) were then placed in medical journals that were read by physicians to influence their prescribing habits in favor of HRT.
- Physicians are invited to conventions and lectures paid for by the pharma companies – often held at attractive vacation venues.
- Physicians are visited by pharma sales reps that leave "free" samples of their HRT products and promotional literature about those products.

Perhaps the most unscrupulous aspect of the relationship between pharmaceutical companies and physicians is that the pharma paid physicians who wrote prescriptions for their products. (228)

Researchers have discovered that pharma have paid more than $2 billion to 17,000 doctors since 2009. You may be able to learn if, and how much, your doctor has received from pharma companies via this link. (229)

Doctors Are Now Encouraging Older Woman To Take HRT????!

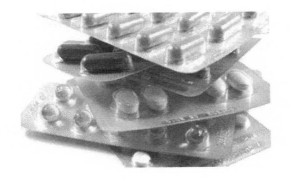

"Stop exhuming the women's health initiative for which doctors prescribe hormones. The WHI for HRT standards is a dead and irrelevant paradigm to modern HRT that needs to be buried."

MARIE HOAG MBA

You may be more confused now .... Than ever before
The North American Menopause Society (NAMS) has just issued a new position statement that endorses conventional HRT for women aged 60 – 65. (230)

The position taken by the NAMS is **reversing** the position of the conventional medical profession on the safety of taking conventional HRT by older women – namely that women over 60 should not take HRT because it greatly increases their health risks. (231)

The NAMS has not stated the reason for its position reversal!

In its statement, the NAMS has not presented any new research that overturns the earlier research that found that conventional HRT should not be taken by women over 60 years of age!

The NAMS statement uses the stale and timeworn phrase "the benefits outweigh the risks" … when taking HRT.

The NAMS has issued their statement about HRT in conjunction with an acknowledgment that:

- Hot flashes and night sweats persist for an average of 7.4 years and for many women more than 10 years.
- 42% of women between the ages of 60-65 have moderate to severe hot flashes/night sweats.

HEALTH RISKS ASSOCIATED WITH TAKING CONVENTIONAL HRT

Conventional HRT can be taken in two forms, estrogen only and estrogen + progestin.

Estrogen + progestin are the form of conventional HRT that is prescribed for most women. But it is associated with known health risks.

Medical studies have found that it increases the risk of breast cancer, heart attack, stroke and blood clots in women who take it. (232)

Furthermore, according to the National Cancer Institute, there can be no doubt that taking conventional HRT increases the risks of breast cancer, heart attack, stroke and other diseases. (220)

These risks are acknowledged by the conventional medical profession because they say to take conventional HRT for just a short time (usually for less than 5 years) and in a small dosage.

Yet most women suffer menopause symptoms for longer than 5 years.

WHY HAS THE NAMS TAKEN THIS NEW POSITION?

As the NAMS have not stated its reason for this U turn, it seems that the NAMS is using its influence to encourage doctors to prescribe conventional HRT for older women, for reasons best known to the NAMS.

I can only speculate about their reason for reversing the position held by the conventional medical profession on HRT for older women, until now.

The position taken by conventional medical professionals until now, has meant that conventional HRT is not an acceptable treatment for a large segment of menopausal women, older women.

The new position satisfies the desires of two influential parts of the conventional medical community:

1. It provides doctors with a treatment they can use for older women, who obviously have menopause symptoms and are asking their doctors for a treatment to relieve them.

    Conventional HRT is the only treatment that conventional medicine has to relieve menopause symptoms.
2. It provides pharmaceutical companies, who make the conventional HRT products, with an opportunity to significantly increase their sales of these products and their profits.

I challenge the NAMS to state its reasons for this position reversal.

Furthermore, menopausal women are crying out for safe treatments to relieve their symptoms.

It is estimated that **only 20% of menopausal women use conventional** HRT, because of the health risks associated with it.

Perhaps the NAMS can exert its influence on menopause researchers to find other treatments that effectively relieve menopause symptoms, without increasing the health risks of women.

A starting point could be for the NAMS to use its influence to bring about a clinical trial on bioidentical hormones.

There are a large number of menopausal women who are taking bioidentical hormones for relief of their symptoms, with excellent results.

There have been observational studies that have found that bioidentical hormones are extremely effective at relieving menopause symptoms, without the health risks associated with conventional HRT. However, there have been no clinical trials on bioidentical hormones!

Yet, there have been spokesmen for the conventional medical community who have warned about "risks" in taking bioidentical hormones, when no risks have ever been found by a clinical trial.

It is also ironic, that these same spokesmen encourage women to take conventional HRT, when clinical trials have clearly found that it increases a woman's health risks.

It is understood, that 75% of clinical trials are funded by pharmaceutical companies and that it is not in their interests to fund a clinical trial on bioidentical hormones. They manufacture the conventional HRT products.

However, 25% of clinical trials are funded by sources other than pharmaceutical companies- i.e., NIH. Perhaps the NAMS can influence one of these sources to fund a clinical trial on bioidentical hormones.

Complementary and Alternative Medicine- CAM

76% of Menopausal Women Use Complementary and Alternative Medicine

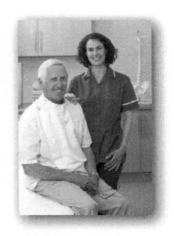

"Mainstream medicine would be way different if they focused on prevention even half as much as they focused on intervention..."

ANONYMOUS

Today there are more visits to CAM practitioners that primary care physicians.

Menopausal women use CAM treatments to relieve their symptoms of menopause. Researchers found that ongoing fear of the potential risks of hormone therapy is the primary reason for the growing use of CAM.

CAM stands for Complementary and Alternative Medicine. CAM is a general term for healthcare practices and products not associated with the conventional medical profession.

Some of the more commonly accessed CAM practitioner groups include massage therapists, naturopaths, herbalists, chiropractors, osteopaths, and acupuncturists, physiologists and nutritionists. The more popular self-prescribed CAM supplements, activities include vitamins and minerals, yoga, meditation, herbal medicines, aromatherapy oils and/or Chinese medicines.

A survey has revealed that 76% of menopausal women use complementary and alternative medicine (CAM). This level of usage of CAM is confirmed by the OB-GYN journal. It reports that 75% of menopausal woman use CAM treatments. (233)

If you are in your late 30s, or your 40s, or early 50s, there's a good chance that you're already taking a cocktail of prescription meds every day for disturbed sleep, mood swings, anxiety, weight gain and other body aches and pains brought about by menopause.

Chances are that you went to see your physician for menopause relief. What happens too often is the physician, having heard a few of your complaints and being pressed for time, probably whipped out the prescription pad and sent you away with one or more prescriptions.

Too many conventional medical practitioners follow this approach. It doesn't have to be this way.

MEDICAL DOCTORS AND CAM TREATMENTS FOR MENOPAUSE SYMPTOMS

Now the conventional medical community is beginning to recognize the role that CAM has in helping woman to achieve menopause relief.

An article appearing in the OB-GYN Journal, (234) says that CAM treatments can help menopausal women and that doctors have to become more aware of CAM treatments.

In fact research has revealed that doctors are more likely, than the general population, to use CAM treatments for themselves. (235)

Today you can have a primary care physician who practices both conventional medicine and CAM. Such a doctor is called a holistic doctor. (236)

CONVENTIONAL MEDICINE ADVICE FOR MENOPAUSE RELIEF

The advice from practitioners of conventional medicine is to take HRT for relief of menopause symptoms, because it is the most effective treatment. But it is associated with known health risks.

These risks are acknowledged by the medical community because they say to take HRT for just a short time (usually for less than two years) and in a small dosage.

The majority of menopausal women do not take HRT; either because they are not willing to assume the health risks associated with it or they can't take HRT because of prior health conditions or family health history.

Less than 20% of menopausal women take HRT to relieve their symptoms. While doctors recommend that it should be taken for a short time – approximately 2 years – many women experience symptoms for 5 – 10 years. If these women take HRT and then stop within 2 years, they will re-experience the symptoms they had previously.

What is a woman to do if she still has symptoms when the two years elapses? It may seem that there are only two options:

1. Either she keeps taking HRT for longer than recommended, in which case she incurs even higher health risks.
2. She stops taking HRT and suffers with her menopause symptoms for as long as they last.

There is actually a third option. She can use complementary and alternative medicine treatments for her symptoms, when she stops taking HRT.

CAM TREATMENTS THAT RELIEVE MENOPAUSE SYMPTOMS

According to the NCCAM (The National Center for Complementary and Alternative Medicine), which is a part of the National Institutes for Health (NIH), CAM involves two kinds of treatments (237):

1. Treatments using natural products.
2. Treatments using "mind and body" techniques.

Here is what NCCAM says about "mind and body" treatments for menopause symptoms (238):

"A growing body of evidence suggests that mind and body practices such as yoga, tai chi, qi gong, and acupuncture may benefit women during menopause. Research is under way to explore these preliminary findings.

A 2010 review of 21 papers assessed mind and body therapies for menopausal symptoms. The researchers found that yoga, tai chi, and meditation-based programs may be helpful in reducing common menopausal symptoms including the frequency and intensity of hot flashes, sleep and mood disturbances, stress, and muscle and joint pain."

The researchers also found that acupuncture may reduce the frequency and severity of hot flashes.

A review of the use of herbal and "mind and body" treatments for menopause relief has been conducted by a medical doctor at the Brown University Medical School. The findings have been published in the OB-GYN journal. (234)

The conclusion reached is that herbal and "mind and body" techniques can be recommended as an alternative to HRT for treating postmenopausal symptoms.

Recent surveys in the United States demonstrate the substantial presence of complementary and alternative medicine in our health care system. Visits to CAM practitioners exceeded visits to primary care physicians by more than 243 million.

Hot Flash Relief: A New Effective Natural Non – Hormonal Treatment

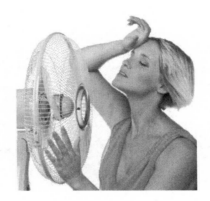

The topic of treating hot flashes, or any menopause symptom for that matter, results in an emotional debate among menopausal women.

There are women who will:

- Use any treatment that will relieve their symptoms now.
- Use only medically approved treatments.
- Use only natural hormonal treatments.
- Use only natural non-hormonal treatments.

Opinions abound. Severity of symptoms varies. Life circumstances vary. Philosophy of life (quality of life now vs future health risks) varies.

What is generally agreed amongst menopausal women is that there is no right or wrong way to deal with menopause and the challenges it presents. The way in which you respond is a matter of personal choice.

This post may be of interest to any woman who is experiencing moderate to severe hot flashes. It **WILL** definitely be of interest to women who are experiencing moderate to severe hot flashes, who are seeking a natural, non-hormonal treatment to relieve them.

A new effective treatment for hot flashes was presented at the annual meeting of the North American Menopause Society (NAMS) last month. Over 2,000 physicians and medical researchers were present for the presentation. (239)

The treatment is called Relizen.

Relizen has been clinically shown to reduce hot flashes. It has been used by over one million women in 13 European countries over the last 15 years. It is one of the leading menopause products in France.

It was developed in Sweden from a purified Swedish flower pollen extract, which contains over 180 nutrients. It has just been introduced in the United States.

THE RESULTS FROM A CLINICAL TRIAL OF RELIZEN:

In a clinical trial consisting of 400 menopausal women that took place over 3 months (240). The participants reported the following:

1. The number of their hot flashes reduced by 26%
2. The intensity of their night sweats reduced by 67%
3. The intensity of their hot flashes reduced by 64%

A survey of the participants was conducted after the trial. Participants said that they experienced:

- 54% reduction in irritability
- 51% reduction in fatigue

- 48% improvement in quality of life
- 47% improvement in quality of sleep

Relizen was found to be completely safe. It did not impact hormone levels differently from placebo (a sugar pill). It demonstrated no estrogenic activity, unlike other natural products that are soy based.

MEDICAL BACKING FOR RELIZEN

As Relizen was only introduced to the United States a few months ago, it does not yet have FDA backing. However it has prestigious medical backing.

It is supported by an expert Physician Advisory Board composed of leaders in the field of women's health....including two prominent OB-GYNs, who are former presidents of the North American Menopause Society and an OB-GYN who is Vice President of the French Association for Breast Cancer.

If Relizen is of interest to you as a treatment for hot flashes, read all you can find about it. If you have a trusted medical advisor, it may be advisable to share information about Relizen with her/him.

How to Sleep Better At Night despite Your Hot Flashes

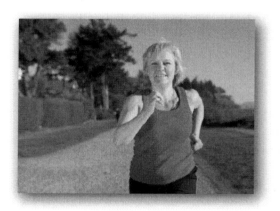

"Physical fitness is not only one of the most important keys to a healthy body. It is the basis of dynamic and creative intellectual activity."

JOHN F. KENNEDY

Hot flashes keep me awake for much of the night...sounds familiar?! Maybe there is a better way to deal with the hot flashes that keep you awake through the night, than putting your head in a freezer!

Maybe the answer can be found in looking for ways to improve your sleep, rather than looking for ways to reduce your hot flashes.

If you are exhausted because hot flashes keep you awake throughout the night, what you really want is a solution that will help you sleep better. It would wonderful if that solution also reduced your hot flashes, but if it didn't and you found a way to sleep better during the hot flashes....my guess is that you would be interested in it.

That solution could be exercise.

There have been many studies conducted to examine the affect that exercise has on hot flashes. To date, the studies have been inconclusive. Some studies have found that exercise reduces hot flashes. Other studies have found that exercise does not reduce hot flashes.

However, the research on the affect that exercise has on sleep is conclusive.

All studies have found that exercise improves sleep quality. Exercise even improves the sleep quality of menopausal women who experience hot flashes. (242)

In March of this year, the National Sleep Foundation released the results of its 2013 Sleep in America poll. (242) It shows a compelling association between exercise and sleep:

- Vigorous exercisers were twice as likely to have a good night's sleep compared to non-exercisers. Seventy-two percent said they never had problems waking up too early and not being able to go back to sleep and 69 percent said they didn't have difficulties falling asleep.
- 67% of moderate and light exercisers said that they regularly had a good night's sleep. More than three-quarters of them said they had very good or fairly good sleep in the past two weeks.
- 76% of the non-exercisers said that they have difficulty falling asleep and they wake up early and are not able to go back to sleep

The lead researcher (243) summarized the results by saying:

"We found that exercise and sleep go together, hand in hand. We also found a step-wise increase in how vigorous the quality is, in terms of how much you

exercise. So if you say you exercise a lot, we found better sleep quality. For people who don't exercise at all we found more sleep problems."

The North American Menopause Society says that just by increasing your physical activity, by doing household chores and care giving activities, you will sleep better. (244)

It would seem to make sense that exercise could increase your hot flashes. When you engage in exercise, your body temperature rises. With a rise in body temperature, you would expect your hot flashes to increase. Apparently this happens with some women, but not with others.

The rise in body temperature that occurs when you exercise is the mechanism that will help you to sleep better (245). Your body temperature will fall several hours later by an equivalent amount.

The fall in body temperature is what allows you to sleep better. If you do moderately strenuous exercise, your body temperature will rise more than if you do light exercise. It will also fall by more, when you sleep.

Here is what Dr. Robert D. Oexman, (246) director of the Sleep to Live Institute, has to say about sleep and exercise:

"Exercise is great for sleep. It reduces the time it takes to fall asleep and increases the quality of sleep. To fall asleep and maintain sleep at night, our core body temperature needs to decrease. You can enhance this need for the core body temperature to drop by exercising three to four hours before bedtime. Your core temperature will rise with exercise and then begin to drop about the time you need to go to sleep. If you exercise too close to bedtime, your increased core body temperature will make it difficult to fall asleep (think about how you sleep when you have a temperature, not very good)."

As Dr. Robert D. Oexman is not speaking specifically about menopausal women when he says to exercise 3 – 4 hours before bedtime, and given the propensity for your body to overheat, I recommend that you exercise in the morning or early afternoon. (249)

If you have had enough of walking around like a zombie during the day, because of exhaustion from disturbed sleep, I recommend that you do 30 minutes of exercise a day. The more you do, the better you will sleep.

12 Solutions to Improve Your Sleep during Menopause

"The night is the hardest time to be alive and 4 am knows all my secrets."

POPPY Z. BRITE

I am awake, but I am not aware. I am functioning, but I am not feeling. This is what Alice said to describe what her life had become, as a result of her disturbed sleep during menopause.

She went on to explain that when she lies down to sleep, her body is ready to shut down but her mind keeps going and going. She said it finds every little thing to worry about.....including worry about a hot flash waking her, once she does fall asleep.

She said that she doesn't fall sleep until absolute fatigue overtakes her mind...and then, more likely than not, a hot flash will wake her within an hour or two. As a result, she said that during the day she is exhausted and she walked around like zombie.

Sound familiar?

If it does, you are not alone. 61% of women experience disturbed sleep during menopause, according to the National Sleep Foundation. (248)

To put this into perspective for you, it is estimated that there are 50 million American women who are currently experiencing menopause symptoms.

That means that there are approximately 30 million American women, who are experiencing disturbed sleep during menopause.

A recent sleep survey revealed that 63 percent of menopausal women struggle to fall asleep and 79 percent have trouble staying asleep. (249)

It doesn't have to be this way.

12 SOLUTIONS TO IMPROVE YOUR SLEEP DURING MENOPAUSE:

1. There is compelling evidence that exercise can improve your sleep during menopause. Exercise even improves the sleep quality of menopausal women who experience hot flashes at night. (see prior chapter)
2. One study found that just being active helps to improve sleep quality and that woman should not be concerned about the type of physical activity they engage in, as long as they strive to remain active. It suggests that doing more household chores will help you to sleep better. (250)
3. There are foods that will help you to sleep better. Learn about them and incorporate them into your everyday diet.
4. Meditation has been found to improve sleep in menopausal women. It reduces anxiety. Meditation is a practice of concentrated focus upon a sound, object, visualization, the breath etc. for an extended period of time. In so doing, your breathing slows down, your stress level falls and you are able to sleep better.
5. Studies have found that yoga improves sleep quality and reduces feelings of fatigue. (251)
6. Studies have found that relaxation therapy improves sleep. (252)
7. Listening to music that you love, and that fits whatever mood you're in, has been shown to lower stress levels. This can help you to sleep better during menopause.
8. A review of 46 trials, covering 3,800 patients, has found that acupuncture is effective at relieving sleep disturbance. (253)

9. The Mayo Clinic reports that "the weight of scientific evidence does suggest that melatonin decreases sleep latency (the time it takes to fall asleep), increases the feeling of sleepiness, and may increase the duration of sleep". You can increase your melatonin level by including certain foods in your regular diet or by taking a melatonin supplement. (254)

10. Serotonin is a neurotransmitter (chemical messenger) that sends signals between nerve cells in the part of the brain responsible for the sleep-wake cycle. Low levels of serotonin cause insomnia. (255)

    Eat foods rich in calcium, magnesium, and vitamin B to help with serotonin production. These include most fruits and vegetables, almonds, beans, cheeses (particularly Cheddar and Swiss), chicken, eggs, fish (especially high-oil fish such as herring, mackerel, salmon, sardines, and tuna), milk, peanuts, soy foods, turkey, and yoghurt. You can also increase the level of serotonin in your body by taking a serotonin supplement.

11. Studies have also shown that valerian, an herbal remedy, has improved the quality of sleep for menopausal women. (256)

12. A recent medical study found that daily supplements of Pycnogenol, an extract from the bark of French maritime pine, reduces hot flashes and night sweats, which in turn enables better sleep during menopause. (257)

If your sleep disturbance is primarily caused by hot flashes and night sweats, please note that most of the above solutions reduce those symptoms as well as disturbed sleep.

When Can You Expect Your Hot Flashes To End?

"Evelyn stared into the empty ice cream carton and wondered where the smiling girl in the school pictures had gone."

FANNIE FLAGG

A majority of my menopause patients have lacked accurate information about when they can expect their hot flashes to end. Many of them expected that they would cease when they reached menopause (12 months after their final menstrual period). Others expected that they would ease at that point.

If you are expecting your hot flashes to vanish when you reach menopause, you may be disappointed.

They tend to intensify during post menopause. According to the National Institute of Health (NIH), the percentage of women experiencing them increases sharply in the two years before final menstrual period and peaks one year after final menstrual period. (221)

During perimenopause, the levels of estrogen are falling, but they are fluctuating. Sometimes they fluctuate at a higher level than prior to perimenopause. At menopause and thereafter, estrogen levels are low....lower than during perimenopause.

Hot flashes are not caused by falling estrogen levels during perimenopause or low estrogen levels at menopause. They appear to be caused when the hypothalamus part of the brain — which has gotten used to higher levels of estrogen for many years prior to perimenopause — sees a drop in that level. This area at the base of your brain regulates body temperature and other basic processes. The falling and fluctuating estrogen levels that you experience during perimenopause, and the low levels of estrogen at menopause and after that, may disrupt hypothalamic function, leading to the flashes.

The drop in estrogen confuses the hypothalamus — which is sometimes referred to as the body's "thermostat" — and makes it read "too hot." (258)

The hypothalamus apparently senses that your body is too hot, even when it is not, and tells tour body to release the excess heat.

The way your body does this is to dilate (widen) blood vessels, particularly those near the skin of the head, face, neck and chest (this is the hot flash). Once the blood vessels return to normal size, you feel cool again.

STUDIES THAT EXAMINED WHEN HOT FLASHES END:

- A study followed 255 women for 16 years – from pre-menopause to post menopause. It found that moderate to severe hot flashes continue, on average, for nearly 5 years after menopause and that more than one third of women experienced moderate to severe hot flashes for 10 years or more after menopause. (29)
- One study of more than 10,000 postmenopausal women was conducted to learn more about post menopause hot flashes. The study collected information from these women for 3.5 years. (259) The researchers found the following:
  - 89% of the women experienced hot flushes/night sweats during the 3.5 years.
  - More women had hot flushes (86%) than night sweats (78%).
  - The frequency of hot flushes/night sweats was 33.5 per week.

- Another study that followed 436 menopausal women from 1995 – 2009 (thirteen years) shed more light on post menopause hot flashes. (221)

  All of the women were between the ages of 35-47 in 1995. The findings of this study were as follows
  - The median duration of moderate to severe hot flushes was 10.2 years.
  - Women whose moderate to severe hot flushes commenced in the early menopause transition stage had a median duration of 7.35 years.
  - Women whose moderate to severe hot flushes commenced in the late menopause transition to early post menopause stage had a median duration of 3.84 years.
  - The most common ages at onset of moderate to severe hot flushes were 45–49 years. For this group, the median duration was 8.1 years.

The bottom line from this study: The earlier you begin to have hot flashes during the menopause transition stages, the longer you can expect them to continue during post menopause.

Just as in perimenopause, the prevalence, frequency, severity and duration of post menopause hot flashes varies considerably from woman to woman.

End Note

Menopause journey is a unique creature and differs from one woman to another.

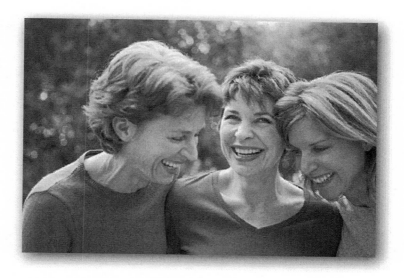

"I can't decide whether I'm a good girl wrapped up in a bad girl, or if I'm a bad girl wrapped up in a good girl. And that's how I know I'm a woman!"

C. JoyBell C.

My own tips to you

ABOUT MENOPAUSE:

Menopause is a unique creature, and so are you. No two women will have the same menopause journey. Start point and end point will vary. Severity of symptoms and their frequency will differ.

The horse racing community has a maxim that appropriately describes menopause:

"Different horses for different courses."

The experiences of women during the menopause journey vary greatly. Some women experience mild symptoms, while others experience moderate symptoms, while others experience debilitating severe symptoms. Some women are done with menopause in a year or two. For other women, it can last for 10-20 years or more.

Also, the life circumstances of women going through menopause vary greatly.

- How old is she when she enters perimenopause? Is she in her 30s, 40s, or 50s?
- Does she have to care for children?
- Does she have to care for elderly parents
- How supportive is her husband/partner of her menopause symptoms? How supportive are the other people with whom she lives?
- Is she employed? If yes, does the job require peak performance for all or a lot of the time?
- What is her personal health history?
- What is the health history of her parents and siblings?

Personal life values enter the picture as well. Is long term health more important to her or is her quality of life now, and in the immediate future, more important to her?

There is no right or wrong, or good or bad, way to go through menopause.

There is only a best way to go through menopause for each individual woman, and that is based upon the above factors.

I believe that each woman needs to come to her own conclusion about the best route for her to take through menopause.

I also believe that it is best to maintain a non-judgmental attitude to the choices made by others, in connection with menopause, and other events in life, because you do not know the circumstances that led to their choices.

ABOUT MENOPAUSE EXPECTATIONS:

The first step in managing your expectations about menopause symptoms and the duration of menopause is education. Educating yourself about the stages of menopause and the phases of perimenopause will help you greatly. This will give you some idea about where you are in the menopause journey and what may lie ahead.

Educate yourself about the all of the various treatments/remedies that can relieve menopause symptoms.

Adopt one of the treatments/remedies that make the most sense to you. If it relieves your symptoms, stick with it. If that treatment/remedy is not working for you, adopt another treatment/remedy that makes sense to you.

Persist and you will find a treatment/remedy that will make your journey through menopause easier.

The second step in managing your expectations is to focus your attention on making your menopause journey as easy as it can be, and not focusing on when it will end.

It is not possible to know when your menopause journey will end. If you keep your attention on when it will end, you will experience increased stress. This will exacerbate your symptoms.

I am reminded of a true story about focusing on an ending, when one has no control over when something will end. The story concerns American POWs, who were held captive by the North Vietnamese during the Viet Nam war.

The most senior POW was an American admiral. He noticed that many of the POWs, subordinate to him, became distraught as a result of setting specific dates by when they expected to return home to the US. When those dates passed, and they remained in captivity, he noticed that they became anguished and frantic … almost to the point of hysteria.

The admiral counselled POWS to keep the thought firmly in their minds that they WILL be returning home … but not to set a date in their minds, over which they had no control.

The same principle applies to the end of menopause for you. Know that it WILL end … you just don't know when. Then focus your attention on making your menopause journey as easy as possible for you.

Allow me to end the journey with the following:

"There is more to sex appeal than just measurements. I don't need a bedroom to prove my womanliness. I can convey just as much sex appeal, picking apples off a tree or standing in the rain."

AUDREY HEPBURN

Bibliography

Fifty Shades of Menopause

1. http://www.drnorthrup.com/estrogen-dominance/

2. http://www.virginiahopkinstestkits.com/cortisolzava.html

3. http://www.theadrenalfatigue.org/what-is-adrenal-fatigue

4. http://www.drnorthrup.com/thyroid-disease/

5. http://www.drnorthrup.com/adrenal-exhaustion/

6. http://www.webmd.com/a-to-z-guides/features/adrenal-fatigue-is-it-real

7. http://www.bcmj.org/article/clearing-confusion-about-perimenopause

8. http://www.ncbi.nlm.nih.gov/pmc/articles/PMC3987489/

9. https://www.sleepio.com/cbt-for-insomnia/

10. http://sleepfoundation.org/sleep-topics/menopause-and-sleep

11. http://www.menopausemakeover.com/2011/06/16/how-to-sleep-through-menopause-2/

12. http://www.aasmnet.org/JCSM/Articles/010312.pdf

13. http://www.johnleemd.com/physiological-effects-estrogen-progesterone.html

14. http://socalbhrt.com/depression-and-irritability/

15. http://sleepfoundation.org/sites/default/files/Summary_Of_
    Findings%20-%20FINAL.pdf

16. http://archinte.jamanetwork.com/article.aspx?articleid=2010996

17. http://consumer.healthday.com/senior-citizen-information-31/
    misc-aging-news-10/menopause-symptoms-can-rebound-after-
    hrt-526792.html

18. http://www.pycnogenol.com/home/home/detail/?tx_
    ttnews%5Btt_news%5D=237

19. http://www.ncbi.nlm.nih.gov/pubmed/15879914

20. https://www.psychologytoday.com/blog/the-athletes-way/
    201301/cortisol-why-the-stress-hormone-is-public-enemy-
    no-1

21. https://www.psychologytoday.com/blog/the-athletes-way/
    201212/the-neuroscience-music-mindset-and-motivation

22. http://www.medicalnewstoday.com/articles/241727.php

23. http://www.menopause.org/docs/default-source/professional/
    news0513.pdf

24. http://www.cancer.org/cancer/news/behaviora-ltherapy-eases-
    side-effects-from-breast-cancer-treatment

25. http://www.breastcancer.org/research-news/20120214

26. http://www.news-medical.net/news/20150330/Investigational-S-equol-nutritional-supplement-may-alleviate-certain-menopause-symptoms.aspx

27. http://umm.edu/health/medical/reports/articles/menopause

28. http://www.ncbi.nlm.nih.gov/pmc/articles/PMC3085137/

29. http://journals.lww.com/menopausejournal/Citation/2014/09000/Risk_of_long_term_hot_flashes_after_natural.5.aspx

30. http://www.bcmj.org/article/clearing-confusion-about-perimenopause

31. http://www.sciencedaily.com/releases/2015/02/150216131117.htm

32. http://journals.lww.com/menopausejournal/Citation/2014/09000/Risk_of_long_term_hot_flashes_after_natural.5.aspx

33. http://www.ncbi.nlm.nih.gov/pmc/articles/PMC3085137/

34. http://consumer.healthday.com/senior-citizen-information-31/misc-aging-news-10/menopause-symptoms-can-rebound-after-hrt-526792.html

35. http://www.iwr.com/becalmd/transmitter.html

36. http://www.sciencedaily.com/releases/2008/04/080421072159.htm

37. http://www.vitamindcouncil.org/about-vitamin-d/testing-for-vitamin-d/

38. http://www.bcmj.org/article/clearing-confusion-about-perimenopause

39. http://www.more.com/perimenopause-symptoms-handbook

40. http://www.34-menopause-symptoms.com/difficulty-concentrating.htm

41. http://raypeat.com/articles/articles/progesterone-summaries.shtml

42. http://menopause.about.com/od/alternativetreatments/tp/Vit_D_Menopause.htm

43. http://www.sciencedaily.com/releases/2008/04/080421072159.htm

44. http://www.sciencedaily.com/releases/2014/08/140806161659.htm

45. http://www.vitamindcouncil.org/about-vitamin-d/testing-for-vitamin-d/

46. http://www.medhelp.org/posts/recovery-after-vitamin-D-deficiency/Some-Impressive-Statements-About-Vitamin-D/show/1359084

47. http://www.neurogistics.com/thescience/whatareneurotransmi09ce.asp

48. http://www.mayoclinic.org/healthy-lifestyle/stress-management/in-depth/stress/art-20046037

49. http://health.howstuffworks.com/mental-health/depression/
    questions/link-between-depression-and-menopause.htm

50. http://www.webmd.com/depression/guide/what-is-
    depression#1

51. https://www.psychologytoday.com/blog/real-healing/201202/
    do-anti-depressants-really-work

52. http://www.beatingtheblues.co.uk/patients/

53. http://www.bbc.com/news/health-20625639

54. http://www.medicalnewstoday.com/articles/8871.php

55. http://www.endocrineweb.com/endocrinology/overview-thyroid

56. http://www.drnorthrup.com/thyroid-disease/

57. http://www.ncbi.nlm.nih.gov/pubmed/15879914

58. http://www.justlaughter.com/ageless_prescription.htm

59. http://www.ncbi.nlm.nih.gov/pubmed/8772471

60. http://www.livestrong.com/article/419079-cortisol-blood-
    glucose/

61. http://www.sciencedaily.com/releases/2000/11/001120072314.
    htm

62. https://www.womentowomen.com/healthy-weight/are-you-
    someone-with-weight-loss-resistance/

63. http://www.maturitas.org/article/S0378-5122(10)00316-6/abstract?cc=y=

64. http://www.naturalnews.com/025301_thyroid_cortisol_body.html

65. https://www.womentowomen.com/insulin-resistance/what-is-insulin-resistance/

66. http://www.cvphysiology.com/Blood%20Flow/BF008.htm

67. http://www.livestrong.com/article/464303-insulin-resistance-hypothyroidism/

68. http://thyroid.about.com/cs/basics_starthere/a/hypochecklist.htm

69. http://www.bcmj.org/article/clearing-confusion-about-perimenopause

70. http://www.webmd.com/women/guide/menstrual-blood-problems-clots-color-and-thickness

71. http://www.everydayhealth.com/pms/abnormal-bleeding.aspx

72. http://www.heart-health-guide.com/increase-progesterone.html

73. http://www.cemcor.ubc.ca/resources/perimenopause-ovary%E2%80%99s-frustrating-grand-finale

74. http://press.endocrine.org/doi/full/10.1210/edrv.19.4.0341

75. http://www.webmd.com/women/guide/heavy-period-causes-treatments

76. http://www.womensinternational.com/connections/inflammation.html

77. http://healthletter.mayoclinic.com/editorial/editorial.cfm/i/163/t/Buzzed%20on%20inflammation/

78. http://www.kidneyurology.org/Library/Urologic_Health.php/Urniary_system_and_how_works.php

79. http://www.mayoclinic.org/diseases-conditions/urinary-tract-infection/basics/risk-factors/con-20037892

80. http://www.webmd.com/urinary-incontinence-oab/womens-guide/bladder-control-menopause

81. http://www.webmd.com/urinary-incontinence-oab/pelvic-organ-prolapse#3

82. http://www.webmd.com/urinary-incontinence-oab/news/20140916/nonsurgical-treatments-suggested-for-womens-urinary-incontinence

83. http://patient.info/blogs/sarah-says/2014/08/female-incontinence-the-last-taboo

84. https://urogyn.coloradowomenshealth.com/patients/library/menopause-urinary-symptoms/

85. http://www.menopause.org/for-women/sexual-health-menopause-online/causes-of-sexual-problems/vaginal-discomfort

86. http://www.healthywomen.org/content/ask-expert/1785/vaginal-atrophy

87. http://www.webmd.com/skin-problems-and-treatments/understanding-your-skin

88. http://www.news-medical.net/health/What-Does-Estrogen-Do.aspx

89. http://journals.lww.com/menopausejournal/Abstract/2014/02000/Clarifying_Vaginal_Atrophy_s_Impact_on_Sex_and.7.aspx

90. https://urogyn.coloradowomenshealth.com/patients/library/menopause-urinary-symptoms/

91. http://www.more.com/health/perimenopause-menopause/your-vagina-menopause-manual

92. http://www.faboverfifty.com/health/the-ring-the-cream-or-the-tablet/

93. http://www.virginiahopkinstestkits.com/estriolhormone.html

94. http://www.healthywomen.org/content/ask-expert/1785/vaginal-atrophy

95. http://www.nytimes.com/2009/03/31/health/31brod.html?_r=1&

96. http://www.ncbi.nlm.nih.gov/pubmed/20109116

97. http://www.webmd.com/sex-relationships/features/sex-drive-and-menopause

98. http://www.sciencedaily.com/releases/2013/12/131204182215.htm

99. http://www.menopause.org/for-women/sexual-health-menopause-online/sexual-problems-at-midlife/decreased-desire

100. http://middlesexmd.com/condition/low-libido

101. http://www.mayoclinic.org/diseases-conditions/sweating-and-body-odor/basics/causes/con-20014438

102. http://www.wsj.com/articles/SB10001424127887323926104578278290520663794

103. http://www.healthywomen.org/content/ask-expert/8989/stress-sweat

104. https://www.perio.org/consumer/cdc-study.htm

105. https://www.dentatususa.com/fileadmin/user_upload/PDF/DentureComfortFastFacts.pdf

106. http://www.webmd.com/oral-health/hormones-oral-health

107. http://www.good-gums.com/menopause.cfm

108. http://www.medicalnewstoday.com/articles/287338.php

109. http://www.webmd.com/oral-health/features/oral-health-the-mouth-body-connection

110. http://www.sciencedaily.com/releases/2007/08/070808132009. htm

111. http://www.oralhealthgroup.com/news/the-sunshine-vitamin-and-periodontal-health-a-vitamin-d-update/ 1000389424/?&er=NA

112. http://www.mayoclinic.org/diseases-conditions/burning-mouth-syndrome/basics/risk-factors/con-20029596

113. http://www.ncbi.nlm.nih.gov/pmc/articles/PMC3570906/

114. http://www.belgraviacentre.com/hairlossinwomen/

115. http://www.health.harvard.edu/staying-healthy/treating-female-pattern-hair-loss

116. http://www.menopause.org/for-women/sexual-health-menopause-online/changes-at-midlife/changes-in-hormone-levels

117. http://www.healthcentral.com/menopause/c/727598/142558/ menopausal

118. http://www.hairdoc.com/hair-loss-answers/chapter-3-the-cause-of-most-hair-loss/

119. http://www.hivehealthmedia.com/research-findings-female-hair-loss-treatment/

120. http://www.livestrong.com/article/135649-progesterone-therapy-hair-loss/

121. http://www.medicinenet.com/breast_anatomy/article. htm#what_are_the_anatomical_features_of_the_breast

122. http://www.livescience.com/1998-breastfeeding-breasts-sag-study-suggests.html

123. http://www.webmd.com/women/guide/a-lifetime-of-healthy-breasts

124. http://www.pmscomfort.com/pms-pmdd-symptoms/pms-breast-tenderness.aspx

125. http://www.2prn.com/breast-tenderness.html

126. http://www.cemcor.ubc.ca/ask/could-i-be-perimenopause

127. http://www.sart.org/FACTSHEET_The_Menopausal_Transition_

128. Perimenopause/

129. http://www.summitmedicalgroup.com/news/living-well/Heart-Palpitations-in-Perimenopause-and-Menopause/

130. http://www.womensheart.org/content/heartdisease/panic_attack_or_heart_attack.asp

131. http://orwh.od.nih.gov/resources/sexgenderhealth/index.asp#h

132. http://www.medicalnewstoday.com/articles/277177.php#what_does_it_do

133. http://www.health.harvard.edu/heart-health/aspirin-for-heart-attack-chew-or-swallow

134. https://www.goredforwomen.org/about-heart-disease/facts_about_heart_disease_in_women-sub-category/statistics-at-a-glance/

135. http://www.everydayhealth.com/news/eight-signs-of-heart-changes-during-menopause/

136. http://www.johnleemd.com/heart-disease-women.html

137. http://www.womenshealthmatters.ca/feature-articles/feature-articles/under-pressure-high-blood-pressure-risks-in-post-menopausal-women

138. http://cortisolconnection.com/ch6_7.php

139. http://heartdisease.about.com/od/lesscommonheartproblems/a/thyroidheart.htm

140. http://www.diabetesforecast.org/2011/oct/how-diabetes-differs-for-men-and-women.html

141. http://www.more.com/health/perimenopause-menopause/prevent-menopausal-joint-pain

142. http://www.mayoclinic.org/diseases-conditions/arthritis/basics/definition/con-20034095

143. http://www.cdc.gov/arthritis/basics/osteoarthritis.htm

144. http://www.cdc.gov/arthritis/basics/risk_factors.htm

145. http://www.medicalnewstoday.com/releases/30060.php

146. http://www.ncbi.nlm.nih.gov/pubmed/20537472

147. http://www.drdach.com/Menopausal_Arthritis.html

148. http://www.mayoclinic.org/diseases-conditions/arthritis/in-depth/arthritis/art-20047971

149. http://uk.reuters.com/article/2008/07/31/uk-britain-joke-life-idUKL129052420080731

150. http://www.menopauserx.com/health_center/health_Gas.htm

151. http://www.webmd.com/digestive-disorders/features/what-are-probiotics

152. http://blogs.nejm.org/now/index.php/uterine-fibroids/2013/10/04/

153. http://www.medicinenet.com/uterine_growths

154. https://www.womentowomen.com/hormonal-health/estrogen-dominance/4/

155. http://www.nuff.org/health_statistics.htm

156. http://www.webmd.com/women/uterine-fibroids/features/fibroid-tumors-what-every-woman-must-know

157. http://www.mayoclinic.org/diseases-conditions/uterine-fibroids/basics/treatment/con-20037901

158. http://www.medicinenet.com/dry_eyes/article.htm#dry_eye_syndrome_facts

159. http://www.reviewofophthalmology.com/content/d/therapeutic_topics/i/1308/c/25170/

160. http://www.healio.com/ophthalmology/cornea-external-disease/news/print/ocular-surgery-news/%7B65c76f16-c790-4585-9d73-28e62903d8d5%7D/gender-and-androgen-imbalances-are-keys-to-dry-eye

161. http://www.news-medical.net/health/What-is-Collagen.aspx

162. http://www.news-medical.net/health/What-Does-Estrogen-Do.aspx

163. http://www.ncbi.nlm.nih.gov/pubmed/10415627

164. http://www.lef.org/Magazine/2008/6/How-To-Look-Younger-Than-Your-Real-Age/Page-01

165. http://www.medicinenet.com/alcohol_and_nutrition/article.htm

166. http://alcoholism.about.com/cs/alerts/l/blnaa26.htm

167. http://www.health.harvard.edu/newsweek/Perimenopause_Rocky_road_to_menopause.htm

168. http://www.sciencedaily.com/releases/2009/11/091119141225.htm

169. http://www.iwr.com/becalmd/transmitter.html

170. http://science.howstuffworks.com/caffeine4.htm

171. http://newsnetwork.mayoclinic.org/discussion/mayo-clinic-study-suggests-caffeine-intake-may-worsen-menopausal-hot-flashes-night-sweats/

172. http://www.mayoclinic.org/diseases-conditions/type-2-diabetes/expert-answers/blood-sugar/faq-20057941

173. http://learn.fi.edu/learn/brain/carbs.html

174. http://www.wmmsurveys.com/Pfizer_Menopause_Report.pdf

175. http://medicalxpress.com/news/2014-05-women-menopause.html

176. http://www.bohrf.org.uk/downloads/Womens_Experience_of_Working_through_the_Menopause-Dec_2010.pdf

177. http://journals.lww.com/joem/Abstract/2013/04000/Direct_and_Indirect_Costs_of_Women_Diagnosed_With.14.aspx

178. http://publications.nigms.nih.gov/structlife/chapter1.html

179. http://www.news-medical.net/health/What-is-Collagen.aspx

180. http://www.realself.com/question/increase-collagen-production

181. http://www.news-medical.net/health/What-Does-Estrogen-Do.aspx

182. http://agefoundation.com/age/

183. http://www.biology-online.org/dictionary/Chronic_inflammation

184. http://www.webmd.com/skin-problems-and-treatments/understanding-your- skin

185. http://www.sciencedaily.com/releases/2012/04/120402162546.htm

186. http://www.preventive-health-guide.com/oxidative-stress.html

187. http://www.webmd.com/404?aspxerrorpath=%2ffood-recipes%2ffeatures%2fhow-antioxidants-work1

188. http://immunedisorders.homestead.com/radicals.html

189. http://www.medicinenet.com/script/main/art.asp?articlekey=47814#toca

190. http://www.medicalnewstoday.com/articles/250570.php

191. http://www.allure.com/beauty-trends/2013/the-allure-aging-survey

192. http://www.arthritis.org/living-with-arthritis/arthritis-diet/anti-inflammatory/cooking-temperature-inflammation.php

193. http://www.icnr.com/articles/natural-progesterone.html

194. http://americanpregnancy.org/getting-pregnant/trying-to-conceive-after-age-35/

195. http://www.womensinternational.com/connections/progesterone.html

196. http://www.lef.org/magazine/2006/4/report_progesterone/page-01

197. http://www.lef.org/magazine/2009/10/Bioidentical-Hormones/Page-01

198. http://www.webmd.com/menopause/guide/menopause-wild-yam-and-progesterone-creams-topic-overview

199. http://www.today.com/health

200. http://www.webmd.com/menopause/guide/hrt-weighing-the-pros-and- cons

201. http://www.lef.org/magazine/2013/11/Surprise-Findings-in-Estrogen-Debate/Page-01

202. https://www.nhlbi.nih.gov/news/press-releases/2002/nhlbi-stops-trial-of-estrogen-plus-progestin-due-to-increased-breast-cancer-risk-lack-of-overall-benefit

203. http://www.nytimes.com/2009/12/13/business/13drug.html?_r=3&scp=2&sq=menopause&st=cse&

204. http://www.medicaldaily.com/menopausal-women-obgyns-un-dertrained-and-uncomfortable-study-finds-245493

205. https://nccih.nih.gov/research/statistics/2007/camsurvey_fs1.htm

206. http://www.webmd.com/balance/guide/what-is-holistic-medicine

207. http://www.health.harvard.edu/newsweek/What-are-bioidentical-hormones.htm

208. https://login.medscape.com/login

209. http://www.healthnewsreview.org/2011/03/guest-post-absolute-risk-not-as-straightforward-as-you-might-think/

210. http://www.reportingonhealth.org/blogs/danger-writing-about-relative-risks-can-lead-your-readers-astray

211. http://www.cfah.org/blog/2012/understanding-risk-its-all-relative

212. http://www.webmd.com/breast-cancer/news/20120306/estrogen-after-hysterectomy-lowers-cancer-risk

213. http://www.nytimes.com/health/guides/specialtopic/hormone-replacement-therapy/overview.html

214. http://www.stoptheclot.org/learn_more/womens_health_faq.htm

215. http://www.webmd.com/menopause/estrogen-replacement-therapy-ert-16198

216. http://www.breastcancer.org/risk/factors/hrt

217. http://www.ncbi.nlm.nih.gov/pmc/articles/PMC2211383/

218. http://www.bodylogicmd.com/research/safety-of-bioidentical-hormones

219. http://www.mayoclinic.org/diseases-conditions/menopause/in-depth/hormone-therapy/art-20046372

220. http://www.cancer.org/cancer/cancercauses/othercarcinogens/medicaltreatments/menopausal-hormone-replacement-therapy-and-cancer-risk

221. http://www.cancer.gov/about-cancer/causes-prevention/risk/hormones/mht-fact-sheet

222. http://www.ncbi.nlm.nih.gov/pmc/articles/PMC3085137/

223. http://consumer.healthday.com/senior-citizen-information-31/misc-aging-news-10/menopause-symptoms-can-rebound-after-hrt-526792.html

224. http://www.sart.org/FACTSHEET_The_Menopausal_Transition_Perimenopause/

225. http://www.drnorthrup.com/estrogen-dominance-a-true-balancing-act/

226. http://www.nytimes.com/2009/12/13/business/13drug.html?_r=2&scp=2&sq=menopause&st=cse&

227. http://journals.plos.org/plosmedicine/article?id=10.1371/journal.pmed.1000425

228. http://journals.plos.org/plosmedicine/article?id=10.1371/journal.pmed.1000335

229. http://www.medicalnewstoday.com/articles/205138.php

230. https://projects.propublica.org/docdollars/

231. http://journals.lww.com/menopausejournal/Citation/2015/07000/The_North_American_Menopause_Society_Statement_on.5.aspx

232. http://www.webmd.com/menopause/news/20070711/hormone-therapy-not-for-older-women

233. http://consumer.healthday.com/encyclopedia/breast-cancer-7/breast-cancer-news-94/hormone-replacement-therapy-new-facts-646066.html

234. http://www.takingcharge.csh.umn.edu/conditions/menopause

235. http://www.sciencedaily.com/releases/2013/01/130110212332.htm

236. http://onlinelibrary.wiley.com/doi/10.1111/j.1475-6773.2011.01304.x/abstract

237. http://www.webmd.com/balance/guide/what-is-holistic-medicine

238. https://nccih.nih.gov/health/integrative-health

239. https://nccih.nih.gov/health/menopause/menopausesymptoms

240. http://www.prweb.com/releases/2014/10/prweb12289158.htm

241. https://relizen.com/Consumer/Real-Results

242. http://journals.lww.com/menopausejournal/Citation/2014/04000/Efficacy_of_exercise_for_menopausal_symptoms___a.5.aspx

243. http://sleepfoundation.org/media-center/press-release/national-sleep-foundation-poll-finds-exercise-key-good-sleep

244. http://www.cbsnews.com/news/working-out-before-bedtime-may-mean-better-sleep/

245. http://www.menopause.org/docs/default-source/2013/physical-activity-sleep-final.pdf?sfvrsn=2

246. http://www.medicalhealthtests.com/askquestion/161/what-happens-to-the-body-s-temperature-during-slee.html%3Cbr%20/%3E

247. http://mountainbike.about.com/od/fitnesstrainingracing/a/Improve-Your-Sleeping-Habits.htm

248. http://www.fredhutch.org/en/news/releases/2003/10/postmenopausal.html

249. http://sleepfoundation.org/sleep-topics/menopause-and-sleep

250. http://www.menopausemakeover.com/2011/06/16/how-to-sleep-through-menopause-2/

251. http://www.menopause.org/docs/default-source/2013/physical-activity-sleep-final.pdf?sfvrsn=2

252. https://www.psychologytoday.com/blog/sleep-newzzz/201210/yoga-can-help-insomnia

253. http://www.emaxhealth.com/1275/treat-menopause-hot-flashes-without-hormones-supplements-new-study

254. http://www.ncbi.nlm.nih.gov/pmc/articles/PMC3156618/

255. http://www.webmd.com/sleep-disorders/tc/melatonin-overview

256. http://www.medicalnewstoday.com/articles/232248.php

257. http://www.webmd.com/vitamins-and-supplements/lifestyle-guide-11/natural-good-sleep-tips-on-melatonin-valerian

258. http://www.nutraingredients-usa.com/Research/Study-leaves-little-doubt-about-Pycnogenol-s-benefits-for-menopause-symptoms

259. http://www.everydayhealth.com/menopause/science-behind-the-hot-flash.aspx

260. http://www.bjog.org/details/news/1375983/Older_women_still_suffer_from_hot_flushes_and_night_sweats_years_after_the_menop.html

261. http://www.ncbi.nlm.nih.gov/pubmed/15981376

262. http://www.doctorsreview.com/history/medicine-woman/

263. http://drmargaretaranda.blogspot.co.uk/2012/10/on-hysterectomy.html

264. http://www.bodylogicmd.com/hormone-articles/the-history-of-menopause

265. https://www.nia.nih.gov/sites/default/files/MenopausepartsAP62409.pdf

266. http://www.nih.gov/news/pr/mar2005/od-23.htm

267. http://sociology.about.com/od/M_Index/g/Medicalization.htm

268. http://www.dslrf.org/mwh/content.asp?L2=1&L3=2&SID=240

269. http://content.time.com/time/magazine/article/0,9171,840627,00.html

270. http://blogs.scientificamerican.com/molecules-to-medicine/drugs-in-search-of-a-diseasepharma-targets-women/

271. http://www.bodylogicmd.com/research/safety-of-bioidentical-hormones

272. http://www.nytimes.com/2002/07/16/opinion/preventive-medicine-properly-practiced.html

273. http://www.jwatch.org/wh201203080000001/2012/03/08/codifying-stages-reproductive-aging

274. https://www.glowm.com/section_view/heading/Endocrinology%20of%20the%20Perimenopausal%20Woman/item/82

275. http://press.endocrine.org/doi/full/10.1210/edrv.19.4.0341

276. http://www.medicinenet.com/hormone_therapy/page2.htm#estrogen therapy

277. http://www.more.com/menopause-stages

278. https://www.nia.nih.gov/health/publication/menopause-time-change/postmenopausal-health-concerns

279. http://www.heart.org/HEARTORG/Conditions/More/MyHeartandStrokeNews/Menopause-and-Heart-Disease_UCM_448432_Article.jsp

280. https://www.apgo.org/2013/PP91.pdf

281. http://www.menopause.org/for-women/whats-an-ncmp

282. http://www.menopause.org/for-women/find-a-menopause-practitioner

283. http://www.news-medical.net/news/20140707/Global-toolkit-for-managing-menopause.aspx

284. http://www.newsweek.com/why-your-doctor-has-no-time-see-you-63949

285. http://www.theatlantic.com/magazine/archive/2014/11/doctors-tell-all-and-its-bad/380785/

286. http://www.washingtonpost.com/national/health-science/a-growing-number-of-primary-care-doctors-are-burning-out-how-does-this-affect-patients/2014/03/31/2e8bce24-a951-11e3-b61e-8051b8b52d06_story.html

287. http://www.whendoctorsdontlisten.com/styled-5/styled-10/chiefcomplaint.html#.VaJ4hPlVikq

Acknowledgement

If ever a book was more a course than an outcome, than this must be it. Throughout the course many people partook, in many momentous ways, to bringing the final outcome into being.

One individual was especially imperative to the progression and its success.

To my editor in chief, my business partner and best friend, Jay Hurwitz, who thrived profoundly hard to turn intricate research and ideas into prose, and presented a writing perspective and expertise that will never be forgotten.

His careful examinations of scientific facts, accuracy, clarity, and completeness, and his on-going efforts and feedback have been exceptional and instrumental.

Ensuring it was the best outcome possible, I am forever thankful.

Contact Info.
Web Site: www.menopausematterstoday.com
Facebook: menopause matters

Made in the USA
Middletown, DE
07 May 2016